EAT BETTER

NOT LESS

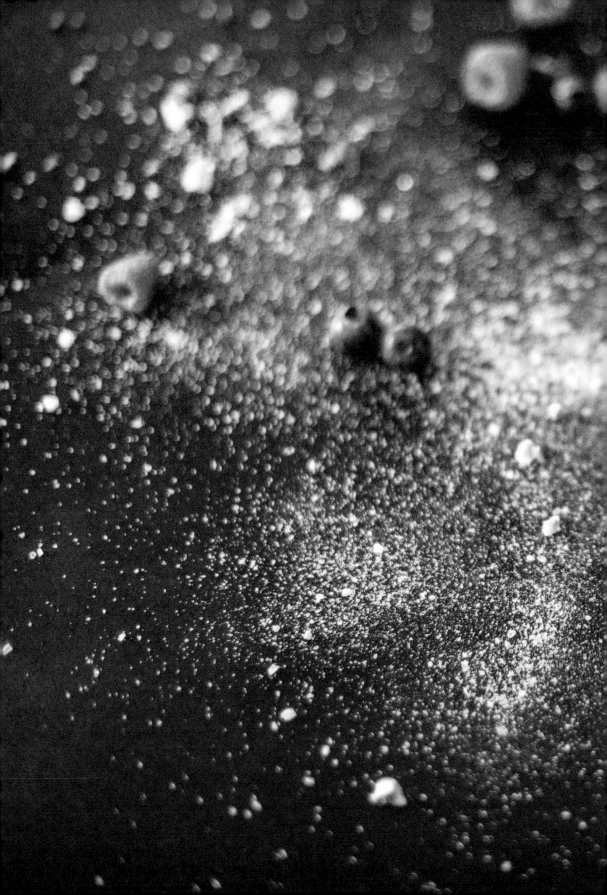

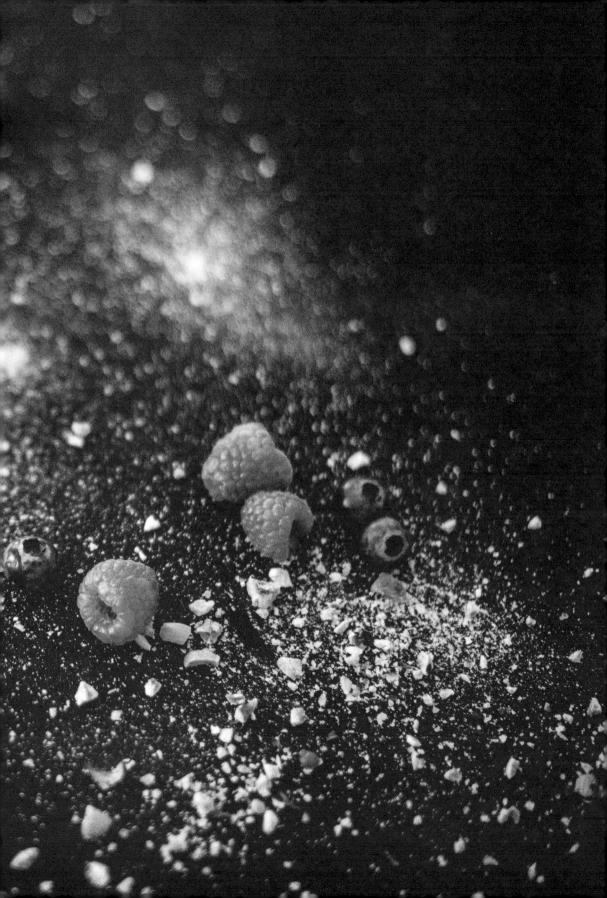

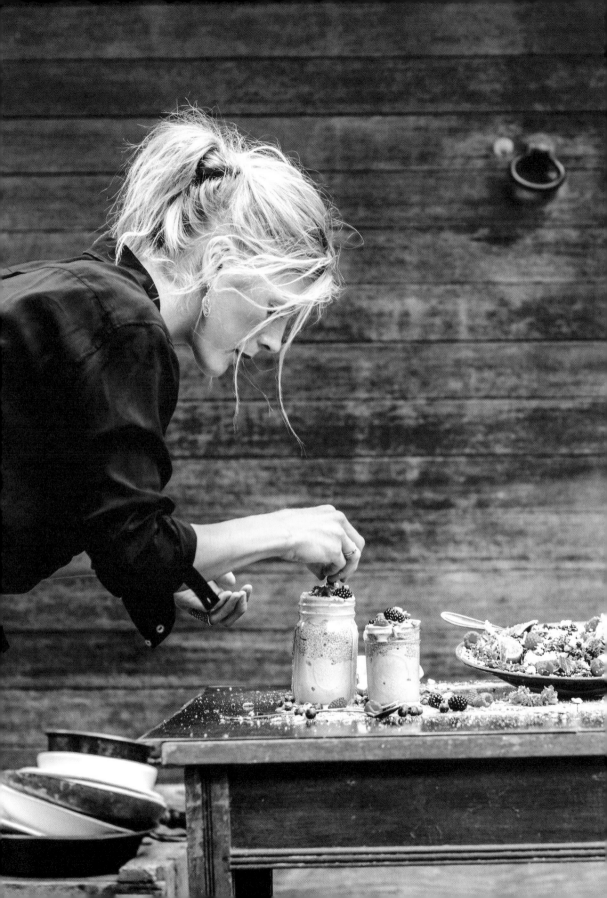

Nadia Damaso

EAT BETTER

NOT LESS

100 healthy and satisfying recipes

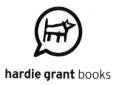

hardie grant books

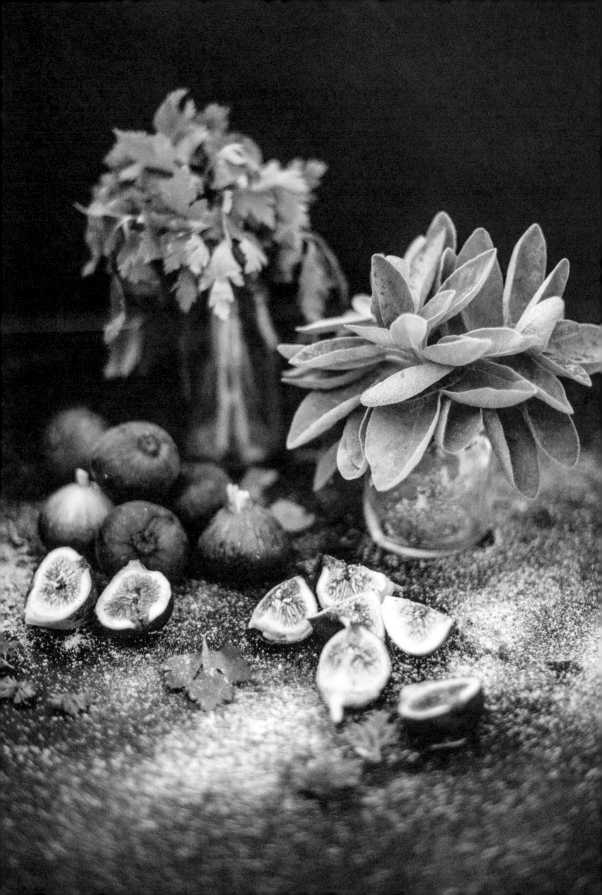

Contents

Recipes

Meat & Fish

Salad & Vegetable Creations

Little Snacks

--- DESSERTS ---

The Classics – Reinvented

Sweet Bits & Bites

Raw Cakes, Brownies, Muffins & Pancakes

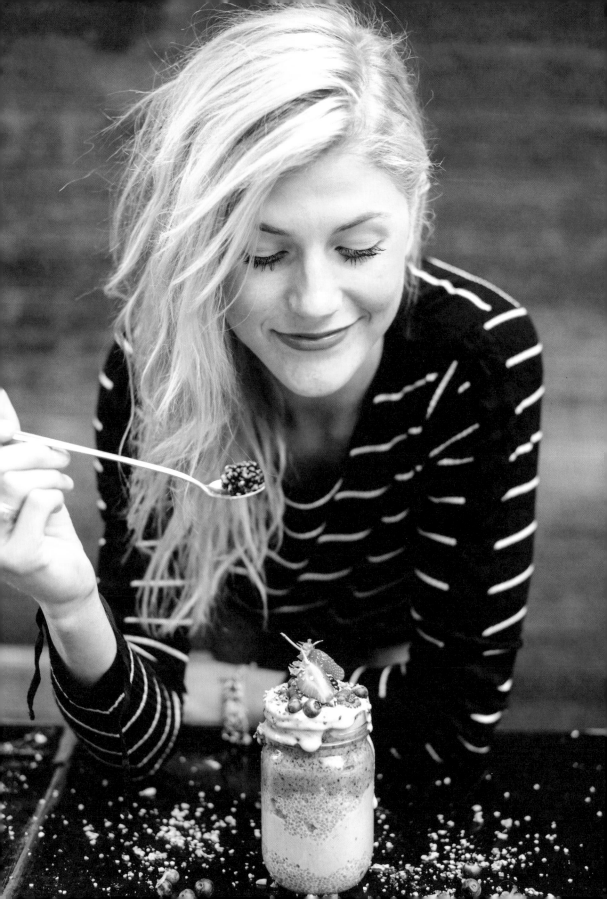

The Book is Finally Here!

I can hardly believe that my book, *Eat Better Not Less,* is finally finished! To get here, I have worked on this book for four months, stood countless hours in the kitchen, created new recipes, experimented a lot and taken thousands of photos. My kitchen became where I lived, but every moment was worth it and I am so incredibly happy to be able to finally share my new recipes with you.

So, who am I? My name is Nadia Damaso. I'm 21 years old and grew up in a beautiful region of the Swiss mountains called Engadin. I'm easy-going and love to entertain people; to give them some happiness from the things that I do. In addition to attending acting school in Zürich, I am passionate about cooking and taking pictures, which I've done since childhood. Cooking is a little bit like acting to me. You can completely submerge yourself in another world, express your ideas in your own way, let your imagination run wild, and put your own personality and character into new, delicious dishes. I love trying new things and I love food. Honestly, good food makes you happy, plain and simple. If you can also share that with friends, family and people all over the world, then it makes it that much more fun! The world is full of different flavours. Every country and culture has its own traditional foods, its unique herbs and spices that bring people together and connect them.

About a year and a half ago I challenged myself to eat more healthily. I was interested to find out how I could cook healthy, balanced, simple and fast meals that were filling, without sacrificing quality and taste. I tried a lot of different things and combined a variety of diverse ingredients. The results amazed me right from the beginning. I could hardly stop; my mind was filled with ideas. Then, without any real intentions, I started taking pictures of my food using my phone and posting them on Instagram.

The photos and recipes were well received, and more and more people all over the world started paying attention and following my Instagram profile. This reaction motivated me to keep going, to create new recipes and keep sharing them. From then on, everything moved really quickly. As I've always loved photography, it was important to me to take high-quality photos. The smartphone camera was quickly set aside and I grabbed my digital SLR that, today, I wouldn't sell for any price! When I woke up each morning I would get so excited about the photos of the new dishes I was going to shoot! Not only is taking pictures a lot of fun, but it's astonishing how much detail a good-quality camera can capture. Sometimes, the pictures bring the food to life so much that all the different ingredients can create a range of emotions. You can see every crumb, every bead of moisture, every piece of ground peppercorn. You can smell the herbs and spices coming out of the picture. That is exactly why cooking, together with my passion for photography, is art to me.

After about three months and another 10,000 Instagram followers I started my first website. I couldn't believe how people from all corners of the globe reacted to it so positively. That response was such an unbelievable motivator to stick with what I was doing and make something out of it. The 10,000 followers quickly became 20,000, 30,000, 40,000, and now, over 150,000 people are following my Instagram account. When you think about such a huge amount of people, you feel very small at first. But eventually you can and should be proud of the work and effort you've invested into doing something you love so passionately that people worldwide have treasured and honoured you for.

A year ago I decided to move forward with everything more professionally. I collected all my recipes and made an ebook that I sold online. However, so many ideas remained buzzing around in my head. One thought that I just couldn't get out of mind was that I needed to create a good and meaningful slogan. Something that didn't already exist. A new brand. The motto, 'Eat Better Not Less' seemed perfect from the start: it expresses exactly what I do. People should eat better, not less. You can read all about my style of cooking and the philosophy behind it in the pages that follow.

I would like to thank each and every one of you from the bottom of my heart for buying this book and, in doing so, supporting my work. Of course, I really hope you enjoy it; that you enjoy the recipes and that the photos make your mouth water. Hopefully I can motivate many of you to try new things yourselves and to create your own unique recipes. Cooking is like art. Sometimes the outcome leaves you speechless and other times it doesn't turn out like you had planned (that isn't always a bad thing though). I am convinced that everyone can cook. It might take a little courage to try something new, like everything else in life. But with a little practice, a lot of passion, imagination and creativity you'll be well on your way.

I hope you have a great time reading and, more importanty, enjoy experimenting!

Nadia Damaso

WEBSITE **www.eatbetternotless.com**
INSTAGRAM **@nadiadamaso_ebnl**
FACEBOOK **eatbetternotlessnadiadamaso**
TWITTER **@EBNLnadiadamaso**
PINTEREST **nadiadamasoebnl**

The Philosophy Behind Eat Better Not Less

Eat Better Not Less will show you that eating healthily is definitely not boring or one-dimensional. I want to show people that if you want to eat healthily, you just have to eat better, not less! Not only is it a lot of fun to eat this way, but it's good for your body and will simply help you feel better. These recipes should inspire and motivate you to create simple, fast, nutritious yet flavoursome recipes that bring colour and variety to the plate. Of course it isn't easy to have a career, family, friends and hobbies and manage to stay healthy, in shape and feeling good without giving up delicious food, especially if you make it all yourself. But, if you're well organised you will see how easy it can be to embrace a healthy and balanced diet and lifestyle. I get asked a lot about what products I cook with and if I have any tips and tricks on how to fulfil the *Eat Better Not Less* philosophy.

WHAT CAN I SAY ABOUT MY FOOD?

I make sure that my recipes consist of 'good' carbohydrates and wholegrains, a variety of fruits and vegetables, and 'good' fats and proteins. It's a combination of fresh, nutritious, good-quality and healthy ingredients that are also illing. As a matter of principle, none of these dishes requires sacrifice because with the right proportions and a little know-how, together with the right delicious ingredients, they are all healthy. My recipes also show that you don't have to give up carbohydrates. On the contrary, the body needs good and complex carbs to be able to function properly. The same goes for the essential fats our bodies need; I only use healthy fats found in nuts, olive oil, coconut oil, avocados and salmon or other oily fish. It's also important to listen to your body and eat if you are hungry. Eat until you are full, not more and not less. Often it's cravings or boredom that drive you to eat when you don't really need to. The body's signals are usually right. As a general rule, you can't go wrong if you trust your gut!

These recipes offer something for everyone. There are dishes for meat-eaters, vegetarians and vegans. There are also recipes for people who love milk products, but the choice of which animal- or plant-based milk to use is yours. The same goes for meat and fish: you can leave it out or replace it with a soy product, or be creative and use a totally different ingredient in its place. You won't find ingredients that don't support this way of eating. These include: refined white flour; high levels of saturated fat; fried foods like crisps (chips) and chips (fries); processed foods that include a lot of synthetic ingredients and sweeteners; white refined sugar; soft drinks and fizzy drinks; canned foods with preservatives; packaged cakes and other sweets and candies; too much alcohol; and ready-made products like salad dressings and sweetened cereals. These foods do not keep you full for very long and do not provide your body with much nutrition – meaning that hunger will strike again more quickly.

Of course, I do not want to force anything on anyone or say that you have to completely give up this or that. Sometimes you just need a pizza or a good plate of Italian pasta. But I can tell you from personal experience that when you take those unhealthy ingredients off the menu for a while and discover which healthy ones you can replace them with, you won't need or miss them anymore. That is exactly what the recipes in this book demonstrate. There are so many ways to make your favourite meals like pasta and pizza, and even desserts, in a healthy and extremely delicious way. And when you really need a piece of chocolate cake or whatever it is that your body is craving, then the 'sin' is worth it and you enjoy every bite so much more.

This way of eating makes me feel better. I have more energy and you can see it in my appearance. I don't believe in diets where you either have to give something up completely or restrict

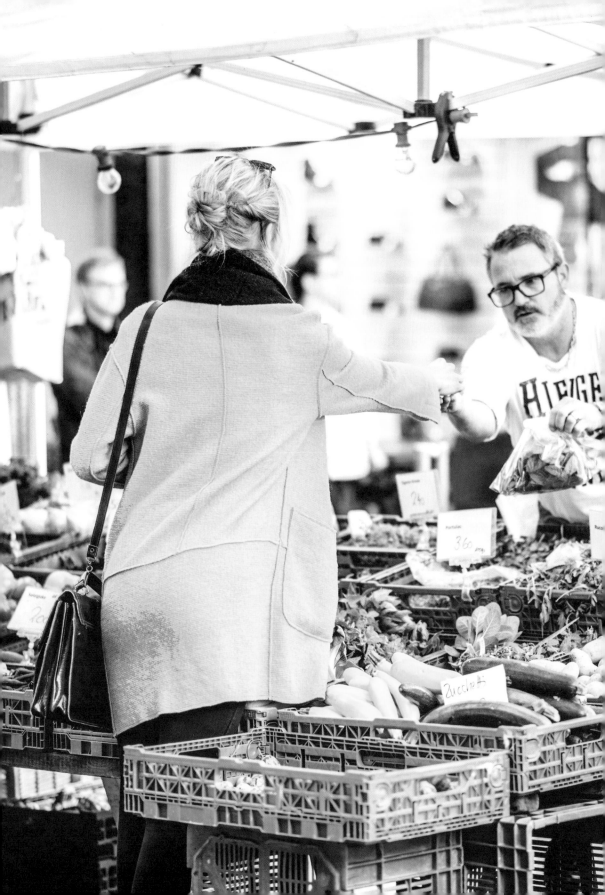

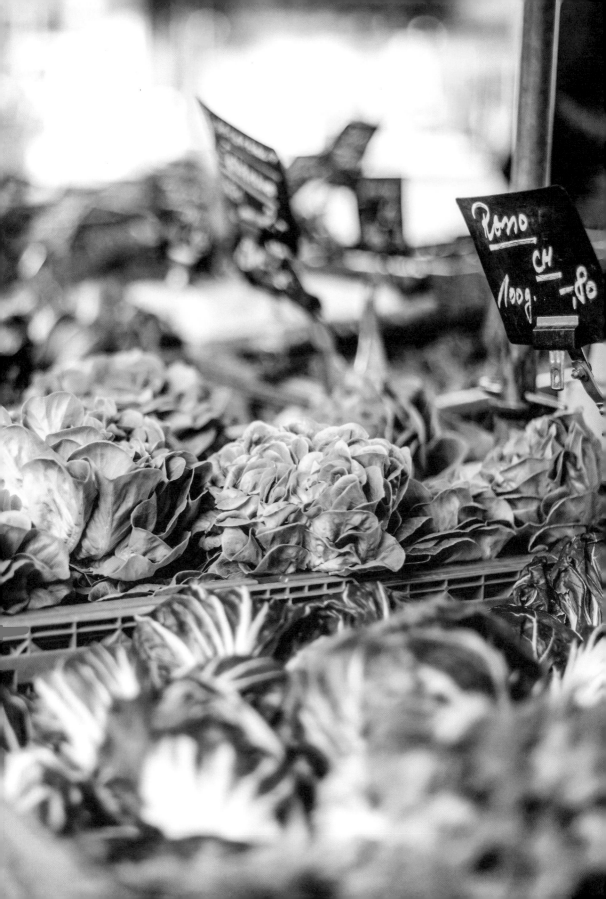

yourself to certain food groups for weeks on end. *Eat Better Not Less* is a lifestyle that opens doors to a delicious world and shows endless ways to create new, healthy and great-tasting recipes. The list of ingredients I use is much longer than the list of foods I avoid.

Naturally, it works differently for different people. You have to play around with the recipes to find out for yourself what your preferences are and to find your own path to making yourself happy and feeling good. If you are motivated to start cooking with some new ingredients, then take a look at my storecupboard essentials on page 20 and you can get started in no time!

WHAT ELSE IS THERE TO SAY?

A healthy diet to me is part of an overall healthy way of life. It is not something that you do for a couple of months to lose a few pounds or 'cleanse your system' or whatever else: it is a lifestyle. A lifestyle in which you have good, healthy, diverse and fresh food that you enjoy and fills you up. And, of course, you should also look for other small things you can improve in your everyday life that are conducive to healthy living.

I'd like to give you a few tips and tricks on how to live healthily, which anyone can adopt. Clearly, everyone is different and we all react differently to certain eating habits and ingredients; some people will digest certain things well and others not so well, some love sports and others have no interest whatsoever... In the end, it's all about finding a healthy balance, but the most important thing is to be happy and satisfied with what you do and who you are.

I'm a huge advocate of breakfast. I could eat breakfast all day long. I love creating a nutritious, colourful, filling breakfast in the morning and wouldn't be able to leave the house without it. You start the day with so much more energy when you have something good in your stomach. Anyone out there who doesn't eat breakfast should try a couple of my breakfast recipes. You will notice immediately how much more energised you feel after a good morning meal. It is all a matter of habit – and this is one of the best habits you could form. If you didn't eat breakfast before, you should absolutely kick-start your day with it now.

Some say that you should eat five to six times per day; others believe that three times is enough. I typically eat three main meals a day and have a piece of fruit or little snack in-between. I personally need an apple a day in the same way other people need coffee. Other snacks for those smaller hunger pangs are things like a handful of nuts, a slice of banana bread, some vegetable sticks with a little hummus, Greek yoghurt with a little honey or simply a piece of fruit or some berries. My recipes are designed to keep you satisfied for a few hours without getting sudden hunger attacks. But if you do find you feel hungry, then a small snack should take care of it. This also ensures that you won't overindulge at your next main meal.

If you try to avoid large portions but always end up coming back for seconds or thirds, try to find a way to feel satisfied with one normal-sized serving. For example, a good trick is to use a smaller plate so you can't put too much food on it. If you're still hungry, then go and get some more. Moderation is the key.

You hear it all the time and it really is the truth: drinking enough water is extremely important. About 2 litres (4 pints) per day is perfect. For a while now I have been drinking a litre of water right after I get up, sometimes with a piece of fresh lemon or ginger in it. It's another thing that you have to make a habit of; I don't even think about it anymore as I do it automatically. The water not only boosts your digestion, but it wakes you up, purifies your body and ensures that you won't have to think about getting something to drink until later in the day. Also be aware that for every hour of exercise you do, you need to drink approximately 500 ml (1 pint) more water.

Creativity and variety in both nutrition and daily life in general are really important to me. Cooking is so much more fun and enjoyable if you always have something new and beautiful to present. Don't be afraid of new flavour combinations. Maybe it'll taste great, maybe not. You'll only find out if you try.

Fresh fruit and vegetables should make up a large portion of your meals. Not only do they supply essential vitamins and minerals, but they also bring colour to the plate, fill you up and taste incredibly good. I can hardly get enough of vegetables. The same goes for fresh, juicy fruit. If you really listen to your body, you can eat until you're full without having a guilty conscience. Extra portions of fruit or vegetables per day is never a bad idea. In my recipes, fruit and vegetables usually make up around half of each dish.

You DO NOT need to give up treats like chocolate, ice cream and pizza. Sometimes you just need it and it's good for your mind and soul! One unhealthy meal every now and then will not make you fat, just like one healthy meal won't make you skinny. In the end, it's all about eating moderate portions and finding balance. It does no good to stress yourself out about what you can, should or must have, or to be constantly counting calories; that stress will steal all your energy. It's more important to eat fresh, natural, good-quality ingredients and listen to your body. The worst you can do is restrict eating or skip meals. That throws off your digestive system, sends the wrong

signals to your body and has the opposite effect to what you want.

Bring movement into your routine: get some exercise. It doesn't have to be an hour a day, but movement does everyone good. It might be that some people will have to overcome some hurdles to get themselves moving more often, but your body will thank you if you do. There are so many opportunities to exercise and find something fun to do, be it jogging, swimming, aerobics or anything else. If you want to achieve something, you just have to be determined, even when it's not an easy path to where you want to go. Whenever you achieve something that you've set your heart on, it will make you happy and proud. And in the end, everyone wants to be content. For me, exercise is the perfect balance to cooking and acting school because I can completely switch off. Working out is like meditation to me. I can go as fast or hard as I want, I'm all by myself and have nothing to distract me except my thoughts (and all the recipe ideas that pop into my mind). You need to find out for yourself what's good for you. But no one has ever told me that they regret doing some exercise. I can only repeat myself: Start to move, I'm sure you will find something you love and will make you feel better. Plus, eating will be a lot more rewarding and enjoyable because you earned it!

When you do exercise and sports regularly, your body also needs a day or two of rest, some quiet time and, of course, sufficient and consistent sleep. If you're mentally exhausted and your body has been pushed to its limits, you simply won't function the way you are supposed to. You will find it difficult to achieve the things you're normally capable of. Just as important, don't forget your social life or pass up on your hobbies. The great thing is, whether it's cooking, eating, exercising, having adventures or simply relaxing, all of it can be experienced with others.

Organisation makes everything easier. Of course, you cannot plan every single minute. It's more about finding the time to cook for yourself or get some exercise. If you leave the house early in the morning for work and don't have time for breakfast, you could, for example, prepare some porridge (oatmeal) and refrigerate it over night. That way you won't have to stress in the morning and you can simply take your breakfast to-go. Another option is to cook double or triple the quantity and store the extra portions in the refrigerator so you can easily take something with you for lunch or heat it up again in the evening. No matter what, not having time is not an excuse I accept for myself. In the end, its just a matter of mindset. My recipes are easy – so easy that sometimes all it takes is mixing everything up in a jar and within minutes you'll have a nourishing, filling and tasty meal. Everyone can get up a couple of minutes earlier in the morning; it is only a question of how strong your will and dedication are to a balanced lifestyle. With some delicious, healthy food you are doing something good for your body in any case.

I always get asked about the cost of eating healthily and all the products I use. I can really only give one answer and it's always the same: eating well and looking good are equally important. If I want to look good and can afford to buy new clothes, that money can also be used to buy slightly more expensive food that will make me feel better. For that, I might have to say no to a new T-shirt or eat out a little less often, and when I do go out I order a water or juice instead of an expensive cocktail. Happiness and well-being come from the inside and you will radiate that energy on the outside. You need to do something to achieve that and believe in yourself. It's all just a matter of mindset and attitude, and it's the same in all aspects of life. If you are motivated and really want something (and when I say really, I do not mean 100 percent, I mean 120 percent), you can achieve it!

Last but not least, remember: eat better not less.

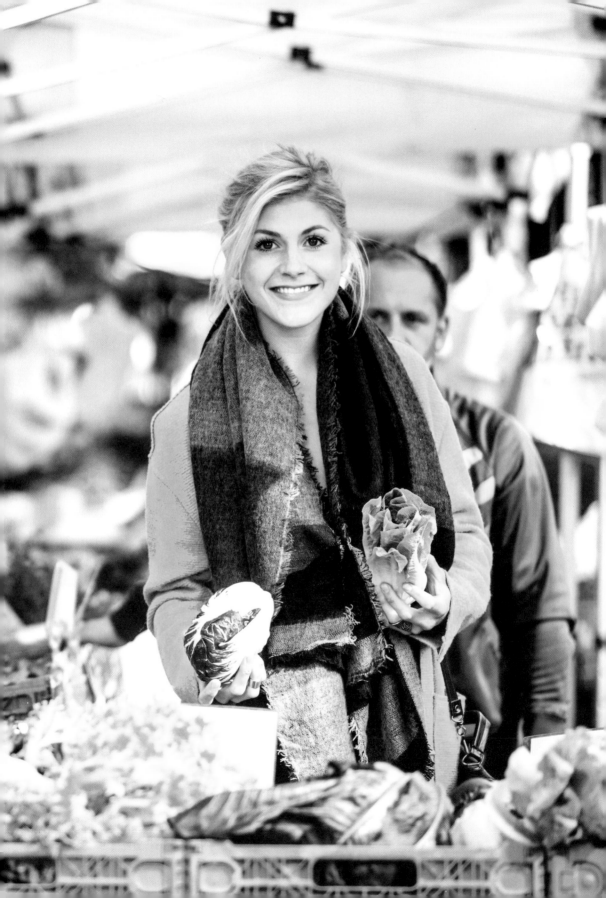

What's in my Cupboard?

The ingredients listed below are what I always have stored in my kitchen and use in my recipes. If your cupboard and freezer are full of packaged, ready-made and sugary products, which are full of preservatives and additives, the time has now come to go grocery shopping and replace them with fresh, nutritious and natural products. Once you have them stored on your shelves, my recipes can then be easily and quickly recreated. Then you will only need to buy fresh produce like fruit, vegetables and dairy products or plant-based alternatives.

Since people are increasingly becoming more interested in a healthy and balanced diet, most products are now readily available at bigger supermarkets at a very reasonable price. If you can't find them there, you'll certainly find less common ingredients or superfoods at a health food store. It might cost a little more, but to me it's absolutely worth spending a bit extra on good and wholesome produce. You are what you eat. The better you feel, the more energy you will have and emit. It's just a question of how much you want it and how strong your will is to eat well and follow a more balanced lifestyle.

GRAINS

Barley: whole, flakes, flour

Brown Rice: whole, flour, cakes, flakes, noodles

Corn: thins, flakes, popped

Millet: flakes, puffed, semolina, golden, flour, milk

Oats: rolled, milk, bran

Rice: milk, paper, syrup

Spelt: flakes, flour, milk, noodles

Wholewheat: flour, couscous, bulgur, bran, tortillas

PSEUDOGRAINS

Amaranth: whole, flour, puffed

Buckwheat: whole, flour, flakes

Quinoa: whole, flour, puffed, flakes

POTATOES, ROOTS & LEGUMES

Beans

Chickpeas (garbanzos): whole, flour

Lentils: red, yellow, brown, green

Potatoes

Soybeans: whole, flour, milk

Sweet Potatoes

Yams

NUTS & SEEDS

Almonds: whole, ground, milk, butter

Cashews: whole, ground, butter

Coconut: whole, shredded, chips, milk, water, oil, butter

Hazelnuts: whole, ground, butter

Hemp Hearts

Linseeds (flaxseeds)

Peanuts: whole, butter

Pecans: whole

Pine Nuts

Pistachios: whole, butter

Pumpkin Seeds

Sesame Seeds

Sunflower Seeds

Walnuts: whole, ground

DRIED FRUIT

Cranberries

Dates: Medjool dates

Goji Berries

Mangos

Mulberries

Pomegranate

OILS

Coconut Oil

Olive Oil

Toasted Sesame Oil

BASICS

Baking Powder (gluten-free)

Balsamic: vinegar, glaze

Fish Sauce

Garlic Powder

Himalayan Salt

Lemon Juice

Lime Juice

Nut Butter

Onion Powder

Oyster Sauce

Spices: chilli, black pepper, ground coriander, cumin, curry powder, cinnamon

Tahini

Tamari/Soy Sauce

Tomato Purée (paste)

Vanilla: bean, extract

White Wine Vinegar

SUPERFOODS

Acai Powder

Cacao Nibs

Carob Powder

Chia Seeds

Maca Powder

Matcha Powder

Protein Powder: whey (isolate), soy, hemp

Raw Cacao Powder

Spirulina Powder

Wheatgrass Powder

100% PURE SWEETENERS

Agave Nectar

Brown Rice Syrup

Coconut Nectar

Coconut Sugar

Date Syrup

Honey

Maple Syrup

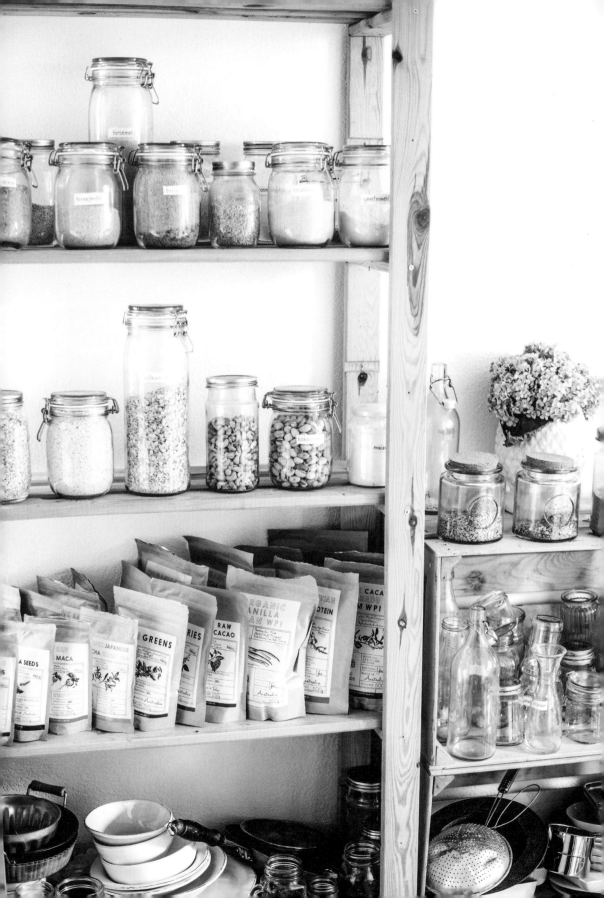

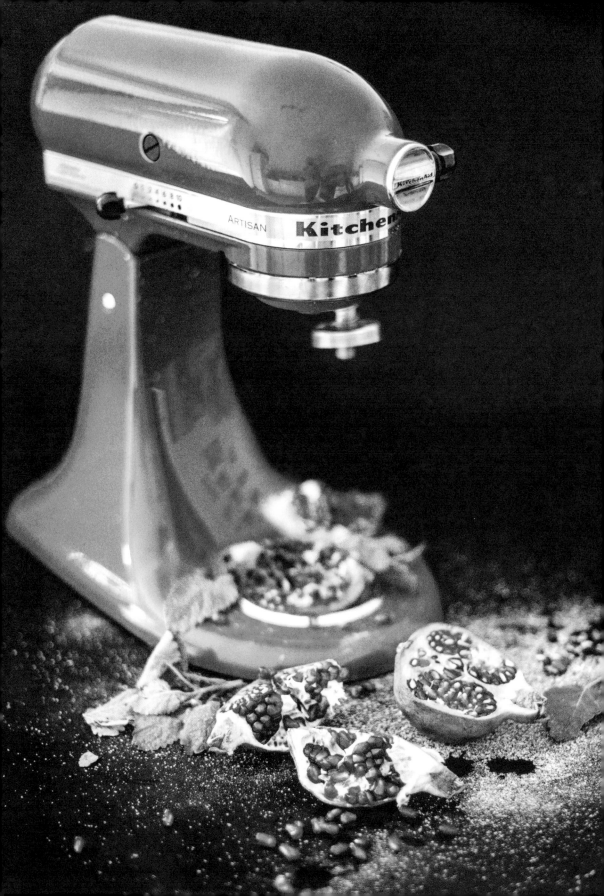

Kitchen Tools, Tips & Tricks

A good blender or food processor is very important for my recipes. Most people think that a good hand blender will do, but the result is just not the same. I highly recommend buying a good food processor: one that is powerful and strong. It might cost a little more, but will last for many years if not forever. With my KitchenAid Artisan stand mixer that can mix, shake, purée, whisk and even crush ice, I always get top results. You can even make nut butter! It's also just perfect for light and fluffy banana ice cream and silky, creamy sauces and smoothies. Almost anything is possible. It is my absolute favourite kitchen tool that I wouldn't give up for anything.

The quantities of ingredients in the recipes are mostly given in tablespoons or teaspoons. I know, different spoons can vary in size, but it doesn't matter that much for my recipes. Simply make sure to use the same spoons throughout a recipe. There is no need to measure out the ingredients in exact grams. A spoonful of the dry ingredients is always slightly heaped and the wet ingredients always completely fill the spoon. The more you cook, the more you get a feeling and sense of proportion. Some recipes mention that if, for example, the mixture or dough is too dry, you can add some more liquid, and vice versa.

Another kitchen tool I always love to use is a rubber spatula. You can scrape everything out of a blender, jar, cup, bowl and glass without wasting anything. I recommend to get both a small and large rubber spatula for differently sized and shaped containers.

Is there anything more annoying than having to work with knives that cut poorly? With a sharp knife, fruit and vegetables can be cut more precisely and beautifully. Plus, it makes it a lot more fun to cook!

Other kitchen tools I use quite regularly are: a vegetable and julienne peeler, kitchen scales, a large sieve, small and large measuring cups, various forks, a whisk, bowls and differently sized pans.

I add a pinch of salt to almost every sweet dish and some sweetness to almost every salty dish. This enhances and intensifies the flavours and makes a huge difference to the taste.

I store ripe fruit in the fridge. What is better than biting into a cold, sweet and crispy apple or having a slice of cold, juicy watermelon? So refreshing!

Keep your fridge and pantry organised and avoid storing things inappropriately. Make sure you keep foods in airtight containers and arrange them so that you always know what you have in stock and what you're running low on. If you can see what you have, you are more likely to be creative with the ingredients you have on hand.

My Favourite Superfoods

Bananas

As bananas are one of my favourite fruits, I believe they belong in almost every breakfast. They're so incredibly versatile. I always use very ripe, almost overripe, bananas. Not only do they provide you with plenty of energy, but they are also one of the best natural sweeteners. It's best to buy a lot of bananas at once and let them ripen for a few days until they have brown spots. It is at this stage that they are at their sweetest and can either be frozen and used for banana ice cream, shakes and smoothies, mashed up and added to porridge (oatmeal), used for raw desserts and much more. Not to mention that ripe bananas are also easier to digest.

CHEERS TO BANANAS

Bananas offer you a real vitamin cocktail: they contain the fat-soluble vitamin E and provitamin A, as well as water-soluble B vitamins and vitamin C. Bananas are packed with many essential minerals, especially potassium, magnesium and iron. They also score well on the glycemic index. If a food has exactly the same effect on our blood sugar levels as glucose, its glycemic index lies at 100. The lower the glycemic index of a food, the longer it keeps us full. Ripe bananas have a glycemic index between 50 and 60.

Apart from all that, one medium-sized banana only contains about 90 calories. Fruit generally contains very little protein and bananas are no exception. However, the small amount of protein that bananas do deliver contains all eight essential amino acids (which can't be formed by the body itself), the most important building blocks of protein and new body cells. Bananas have a very low fat content; this fat is also very valuable because it contains essential polyunsaturated fatty acids. Bananas are simply one of the best, most nourishing and energising foods.

Banana Ice Cream
Creamy, Light, Delicious and Healthy

———— BASIC RECIPE (1 SERVING) ————

2 very ripe bananas, sliced (approx. 250–300 g/9–10½ oz)

100–120 ml (3½–4 fl oz) milk of choice, e.g. soy, almond, rice milk

1–2 teaspoons maple syrup or sweetener of choice (optional)

Optional additions: fruit of choice, vanilla extract, cinnamon, raw cacao powder, dates, oats, protein powder, maca, wheatgrass, berries, nut butters, cacao nibs

1. Put the sliced bananas into freezer bags and freeze overnight or for at least 2–3 hours.

2. Take the frozen banana slices out of the freezer and let them thaw for about 5 minutes. Add to a blender with only a dash of milk at first and blend. To get a smooth, creamy consistency you might have to add another splash of milk. Give it a quick stir with a spoon to make sure all the banana slices are blended in well.

3. Add in any extra flavours you like and blend for another minute or so. Pour into a bowl or jar and serve with your toppings of choice, or freeze (see note below).

NOTE The quantity of milk you add always depends on the size and ripeness of the bananas. Some don't need any milk at all, some do. I like to add a little bit more (usually soy milk) because it makes the ice cream lighter and creamier. Banana ice cream is always best made and eaten fresh. If you want to make it in advance, though, prepare it the exact same way, then transfer into a bowl and freeze. Thaw for 5–8 minutes before serving.

BLENDER It's really important to use a good blender or food processor to make creamy, light and fluffy banana ice cream. In most cases a hand blender is not powerful enough and you will need to add too much liquid. If a hand blender is the only gadget you have available, let the banana slices thaw for a few more minutes and only add about half of the liquid you think you'll need.

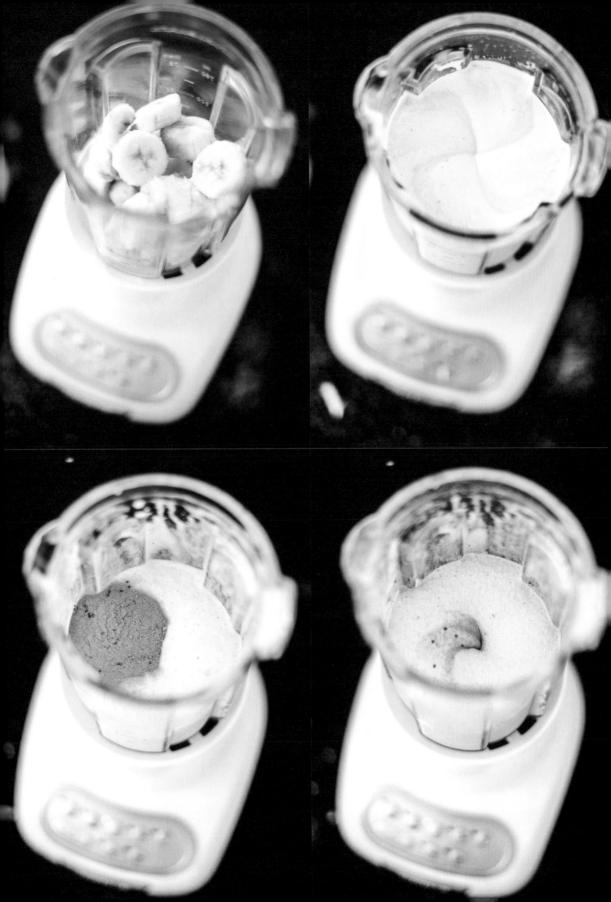

Chia Seeds

These seeds come from a type of mint plant originally from Mexico and Guatemala. Mayans and Aztecs loved them because they're nourishing and fill you up. Chia seeds have been available in shops for a few years now and are sold as a superfood. Chia seeds consist of about 40 percent chia oil (of which more than 80 percent comprises unsaturated fatty acids), 20 percent protein and around 40 percent carbohydrates. The seeds contain vitamin A and B-vitamins (niacin, thiamine, riboflavin, folic acid), and the minerals calcium, phosphorus, potassium, zinc and iron, as well as antioxidants. The fibre content is responsible for the gloopy consistency of soaked chia seeds.

Black and white chia seeds both have a neutral flavour and are very versatile. They can be added to porridge, as a topping for smoothies and banana ice cream, be sprinkled on salads or be turned into chia pudding by soaking the seeds until they have a jelly-like consistency.

Coconut

I absolutely love coconut. You can buy coconuts whole, dried and shredded, and in the forms of coconut flour, milk, water, oil, sugar and nectar. Fresh coconuts are rich in potassium, iron and copper.

Coconut Oil contains only saturated fatty acids. These are generally regarded as unhealthy and are less recommended than monounsaturated and polyunsaturated fatty acids, as they raise bad cholesterol (LDL cholesterol). But because 50 percent of the saturated fatty acids in coconut is made up of lauric acid, which can increase good cholesterol (HDL cholesterol), a balance between good and bad cholesterol can be achieved.

The oil also strengthens the immune system to fight bacteria and viruses.

Like any other oil, coconut oil can be used for cooking and baking. It's also a very good substitute for butter in frozen desserts or home-made chocolate. Many swear by coconut oil for skin and hair care: it cools and moisturises. At room temperature it's soft and spreadable, in the fridge it sets and at higher temperatures it's liquid.

Coconut Flour is gluten-free. It's made from pressed coconut pulp (after oil extraction), which is first dried and then ground. It's rich in proteins, minerals and trace elements. Coconut flour keeps you full and satisfied. Flour mixes can contain 20–25 percent coconut flour.

Coconut Water comes from the inside of young coconuts. In ripe fruits the water is stored in the flesh. Coconut water is rich in minerals (magnesium, calcium, potassium, phosphorus, selenium and iron). The water is very popular among athletes due to its isotonic nature and the associated optimum supply of fluids.

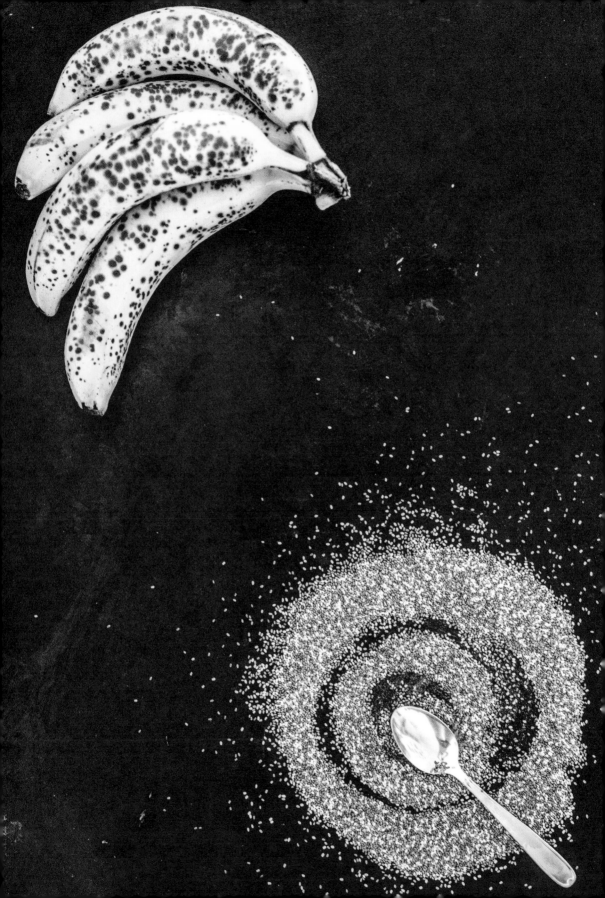

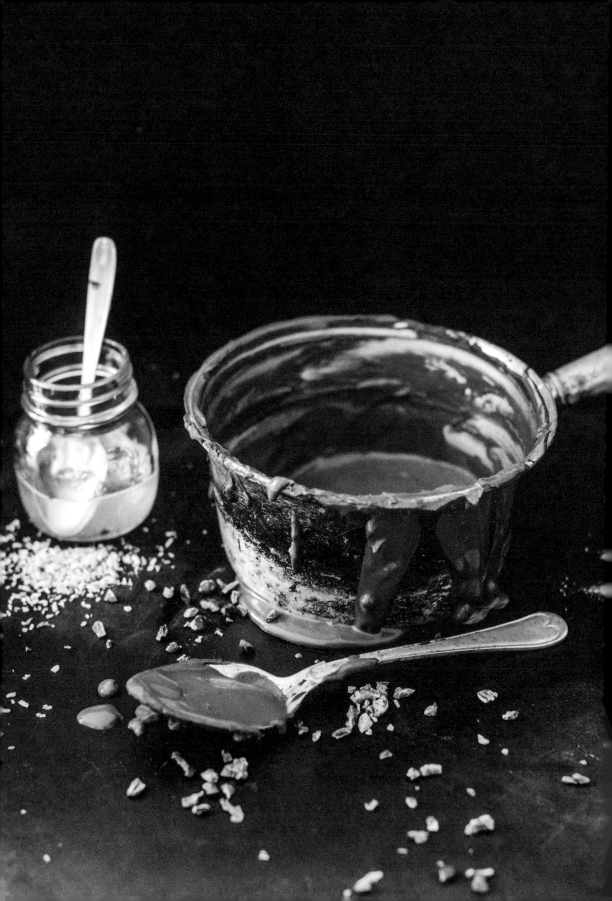

Coconut Milk is extracted from the pulp of the coconut. The coconut meat is grated and then enriched with water, which is later pressed and filtered. A dash of coconut milk can be used to make many dishes and smoothies creamier. It should not be confused with coconut cream, which is thicker and contains much more fat.

Coconut Sugar comes from the sap of the coconut palm flower buds, which is cooked into syrup and then crystallised. The colour of the sugar can vary depending on the cooking time. From coarse to as fine as icing (confectioner's) sugar, coconut sugar is available in different consistencies. It has a slight caramel flavour, is a great substitute for cane sugar and a great natural sweetener in general.

Coconut Nectar comes from the coconut palm and is the by-product of coconut sugar.

Raw Cacao Powder

When I hear the word chocolate, my heart immediately starts to beat faster! Chocolate available in stores is usually made of cocoa mass, cocoa butter, refined sugar and additives. Milk chocolate also contains milk powder. Dark chocolate is the healthier option to go for due to its high cocoa content and lower sugar content. You can also enjoy the irresistible taste of chocolate by making the chocolate yourself, without any refined sugar and additives in it. With only three ingredients, you can make incredibly delicious chocolate and truffles. The secret ingredients are raw cacao powder, a natural sweetener and coconut oil.

Raw cacao powder is made of ground and sifted cacao beans, which have been fermented and roasted. The cacao butter is then pressed out of the cacao mass. Depending on the pressure, the fat content is between 10–20 percent. Raw cacao powder has a strong, distinctive taste. It is very versatile and is used in many of my recipes, especially breakfasts and desserts.

Raw cacao powder is not only full of antioxidants, it's also rich in vitamins and minerals: magnesium relaxes the muscles, calcium and iron are good for skin, hair and nails, and phosphorus strengthens teeth. Besides pain-relieving substances, cacao also stimulates the production of endorphins, which boost the mood.

ATTENTION Raw cacao powder is not to be confused with cocoa powder or chocolate powder. Raw cacao powder is the purest form of chocolate you can consume and is much less processed than cocoa powder or chocolate bars. Chocolate powder is produced by grinding up chocolate and contains refined sugar. I only use raw cacao powder. It costs more than normal cocoa powder from the supermarket, but it's higher in quality and is a lot more intense in flavour. Because of this, you need to use less powder so the high price is balanced out. It follows that the less oil the powder contains, the healthier and more expensive it is.

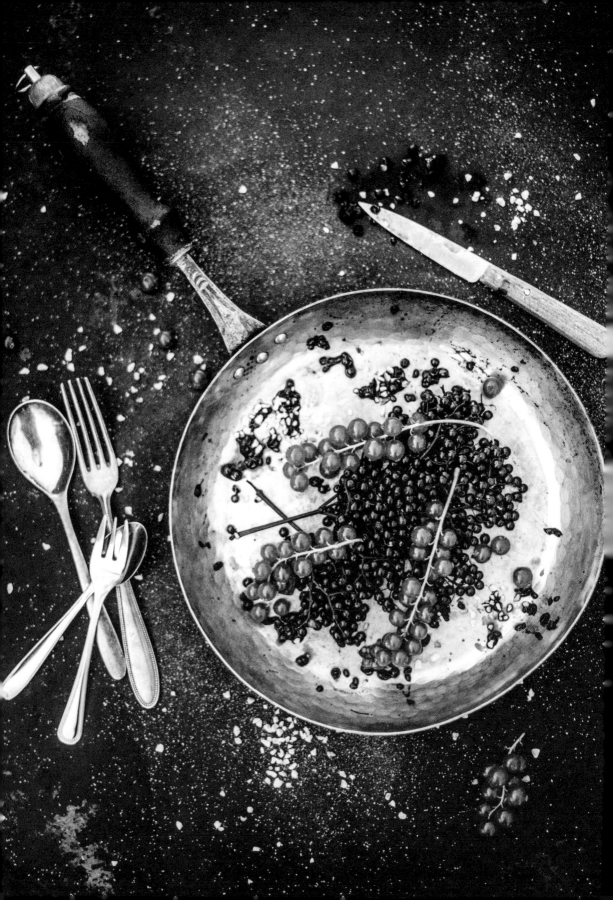

Berries

In my recipes, I often use all kinds of berries. They bring so much colour and freshness to almost every dish. Of course, they're best fresh, but if they're not in season, frozen berries can be used for most of the recipes as well. Berries are packed with vitamins, antioxidants and minerals, are very low in calories and a good snack in between main meals. My favourite kinds are blueberries, raspberries, strawberries, blackberries and acai.

Maca Powder

Maca powder is hailed as a superfood and comes from the maca root, which is dried and then ground into a fine powder. It contains a lot of protein, minerals and vitamins, and about a teaspoon a day added to your breakfast, shakes, smoothies or baked goods can support your health. Maca powder has a pretty strong, unique taste that I personally loved from the moment I tried it.

Hemp Hearts

Hemp hearts are shelled hemp seeds, are high in omega-6 and omega-3 fatty acids and are suitable for those who don't tolerate gluten, sugar or nuts. They have a slightly nutty flavour and are incredibly delicious when sprinkled on salads, in your granola, on banana ice cream or other sweet and savory dishes. From hemp seeds, which look similar to buckwheat, you can make hemp hearts, hemp butter, hemp milk, hemp oil and even hemp protein powder. I use hemp hearts the most as I absolutely love both their texture and taste. They're so nourishing, great as a garnish and give extra flavour and life to your dishes.

Oats

Oats are one of my favourite ingredients to use in my breakfasts. Whether they're cooked into porridge (oatmeal), baked, mixed into smoothies or added to granola, they're tasty and keep you full and energised! They taste even better when combined with a variety of fruit and nuts. Oats contain a lot of fibre and protein, are very low in fat and stabilise your blood pressure. They are available in different sizes and can also be bought gluten-free (which I use in most of my recipes).

Quinoa

Quinoa is one of the most nutritious foods ever! Particularly noteworthy is its protein, which in contrast to grain protein contains all the essential amino acids. For people who can't eat meat, dairy and animal products, quinoa is a great substitute. Just like oats, quinoa is very low in fat and high in protein. The gluten-free pseudograin is a new superfood everyone is crazy about. It tastes just as good in sweet as in savoury dishes.

Millet

Millet has a slightly sweet, nutty flavour and is definitely one of my favorite grains. Out of all the grains, millet is the one with the highest iron content. It also contains a lot of silicic acid (silica), which is why it's also called the beauty grain. Silica strengthens hair, nails, connective tissue and is important for good dental health. Millet contains a great range of B vitamins, which is highly beneficial. It is one of the most digestible grains and can be used for sweet and savoury dishes. It's also gluten-free.

Tahini

Tahini is a seed butter made from sesame seeds. In comparison to nut butter, it doesn't necessarily have to be home-made because it's almost always available as a 100% pure product. Due to its intense taste, it doesn't taste as good as other nut butters when eaten pure, but adding tahini to sauces, savoury dishes, shakes or smoothies, makes magic happen. Tahini adds so much flavour and makes everything creamier. Sesame seeds, white or black, contain magnesium, calcium, iron and B vitamins. It's best to always have some tahini in your kitchen.

Dates

Due to their high energy content, dates are also known as the 'bread of the desert'. Dates are incredibly versatile, contain numerous easily digestible sugars and are ideal to use as a natural sweetener for many dishes. The Medjool date is the queen of dates due to its size. It's also sweeter and moister than the smaller dates and easier to blend.

Nuts & Seeds

Nuts are one of the best sources of healthy fats. Although they're high in calories, they provide a lot of valuable nutrients and are delicious! Whenever I buy nuts, I buy a variety in large packages that I roast all at once and then store in my cupboard. Roasted nuts taste so much better. They're crunchier and their flavour is intensified. Buy unsalted and preferably also unroasted nuts as they're usually roasted with additional oil. I love to add some crushed nuts on top of my breakfasts, salads and other dishes too. Also, I make home-made nut butter to add into things like smoothies and sauces to make them creamier and more flavouful. Nuts are just an amazing, natural and extremely versatile food. A good handful of nuts a day or a tablespoon of your favourite nut butter is enough to cover your daily good fat intake. Nuts contain many valuable nutrients and are a great snack for between meals to keep hunger at bay.

NUTRITIONAL INFORMATION
PER 100 G/3½ OZ

Almonds 569 kcal/2381 kJ | vitamins B2 and E, niacin, zinc, magnesium, manganese, potassium, calcium

Cashews 568 kcal/2377 kJ | vitamins A and B1, magnesium, copper, iron

Coconuts 342kcal/1431 kJ | potassium, iron, manganese

Hazelnuts 636 kcal/2661 kJ | vitamins A, B1, B2 and C, potassium, calcium, magnesium, manganese, copper, phosphorus

Peanuts 561 kcal/2347 kJ | vitamins A, B1 and B2, niacin, folic acid, magnesium, manganese, potassium, phosphorus, iron, calcium

Pecans 692 kcal/2895 kJ | vitamins B1 and E, copper, magnesium, manganese, zinc

Pine Nuts 575 kcal/2406 kJ | vitamins B1 and E, phosophorus, iron, magnesium, manganese

Pistachios 574 kcal/2402 kJ | vitamin B1, calcium, iron, magnesium

Sesame Seeds 573 kcal/2397 kJ | vitamin B1, sodium, potassium, calcium, magnesium, irone

Sunflower Seeds 596 kcal/2494 kJ | B vitamins, magnesium, phosphorus

Walnuts 654 kcal/2736 kJ | vitamins A, B1, B2 and C, folic acid, magnesium, manganese, copper

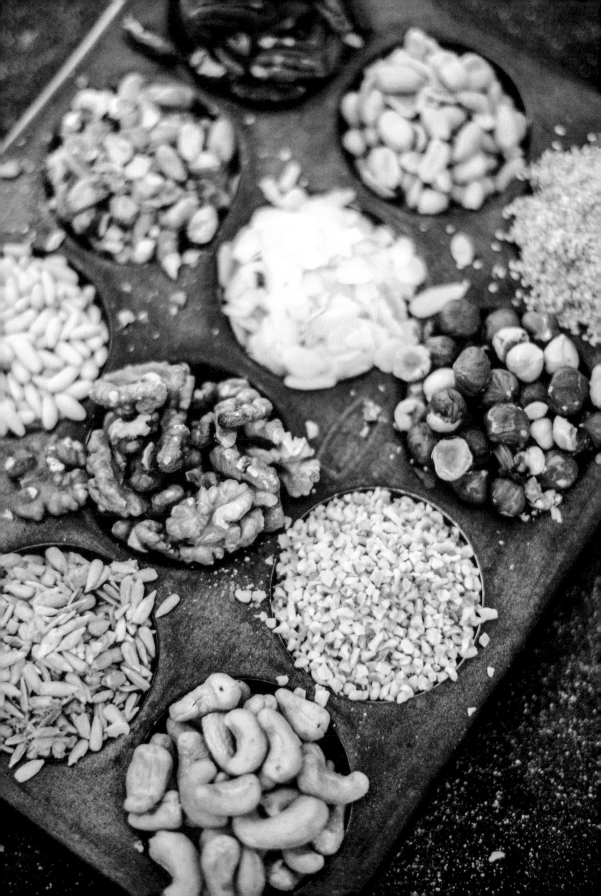

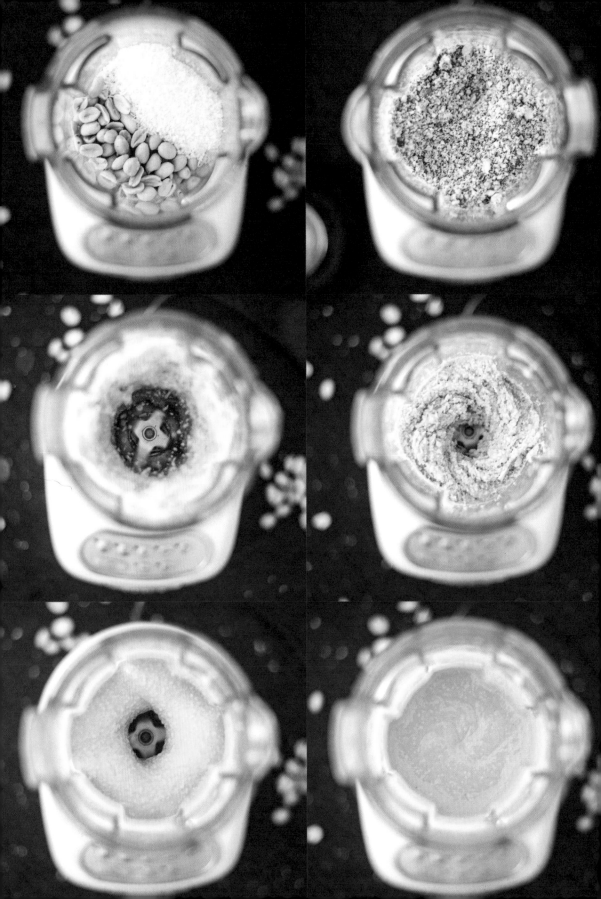

Home-made, Smooth & Creamy Nut Butters

Flipping through my recipes, you will quickly notice that I frequently use nut butter. It's incredibly easy and fast to make and can be adjusted according to your personal taste. It contains healthy fats and provides an irresistibly nutty and delicious note to almost every dish – sweet or savoury.

The most common nut butter known to all of you is probably peanut butter. It's available at every supermarket but usually contains additional oils, refined sugar, additives and preservatives. In health food stores you will find pure nut butter of all kinds without such additives. However, shop-bought pure nut butters can be quite expensive, so I advise you to make nut butters yourself. All you need is a good blender or food processor. Of course, you can add different flavours like vanilla or cinnamon and/or a natural sweetener like honey at the end, but the basic recipe contains nuts and nuts alone. Nut butter can be made with a wide variety of nuts. If you're allergic to nuts, you can use sunflower, pumpkin or sesame seeds and make seed butter instead.

Peanut Butter

_____ CLASSIC PEANUT BUTTER _____
MAKES ABOUT 400 G (14 OZ)

400 g (14 oz) unsalted peanuts, roasted
pinch of salt
1–2 tablespoons sweetener of choice (optional)

1   Preheat the oven to 160°C (320°F/Gas 3). Place the peanuts on a baking tray lined with parchment paper and roast for about 15–20 minutes. Take the nuts out of the oven and leave them to cool.

2   Add the cooled nuts and the salt into a powerful blender or food processor and pulse until they are coarsely ground.

3   Blend on a medium speed for 3–4 minutes. The oils will be released and the mixture will become smoother. Scrape down the sides from time to time to ensure all the nuts are well blended.

4   Continue blending for another 4–5 minutes, depending on how good and strong your blender or processor is. The longer you blend the creamier it gets. With my KitchenAid blender the whole process to an incredibly smooth and creamy nut butter only takes about 5 minutes.

5   Pour the nut butter into an airtight jar. The butter can be stored for up to 3–4 weeks. Make sure that the jar is always tightly sealed.

If you want to add a slight sweet touch, do this at the very end. With a spoon, stir in some of your sweetener of choice. Don't be tempted to blend the sweetener or additional flavours as this can quickly lead to a clumpier consistency.

VARIATIONS   You can make many different varieties of nut butter. You will find a few of my favourite nut butter recipes on the following page.

IMPORTANT   If you want to get a really nutty taste, make sure to always roast the nuts before blending them. If you don't have a lot of time, you can buy roasted nuts. Make sure they don't contain any salt, preservatives or added oils.

Different Kinds of Nut Butters

ALMOND BUTTER

300 g (10½ oz) blanched almonds

pinch of salt

1 tablespoon maple syrup or sweetener of choice

PEANUT & COCONUT BUTTER

200 g (7 oz) peanuts

100 g (3½ oz) shredded coconut

pinch of salt

1 tablespoon maple syrup or sweetener of choice
(optional)

ALMOND & CASHEW BUTTER

150 g (5 oz) blanched almonds

150 g (5 oz) cashews

pinch of salt

1 tablespoon maple syrup or sweetener of choice
(optional)

ALMOND & CINNAMON BUTTER

300 g (10½ oz) almonds

pinch of salt

2 teaspoons ground cinnamon

2 tablespoons maple syrup or sweetener of choice
(optional)

PISTACHIO & COCONUT BUTTER

200 g (7 oz) pistachios

100 g (3½ oz) shredded coconut

pinch of salt

1 tablespoon maple syrup or sweetener of choice
(optional)

COCONUT BUTTER

300 g (10½ oz) shredded coconut

pinch of salt

1 teaspoon pure vanilla extract

1 tablespoon maple syrup or sweetener of choice
(optional)

PECAN & MACADAMIA BUTTER

200 g (7 oz) pecans

100 g (3½ oz) macadamia nuts

pinch of salt

some pure vanilla extract

1 tablespoon maple syrup or sweetener of choice
(optional)

CHOCOLATE & HAZELNUT BUTTER

250 g (9 oz) hazelnuts

pinch of salt

4 tablespoons raw cacao powder

12–14 dates, cooked until soft, or 6–7 Medjool dates

200 ml (7 fl oz) almond or oat milk

1 teaspoon vanilla extract

1 tablespoon rice malt syrup (for some extra sweetness)

How to make nut butter step by step: see recipe on
page 35.

NOTE: I always add a pinch of salt to intensify
the flavour, especially when adding sweetener.

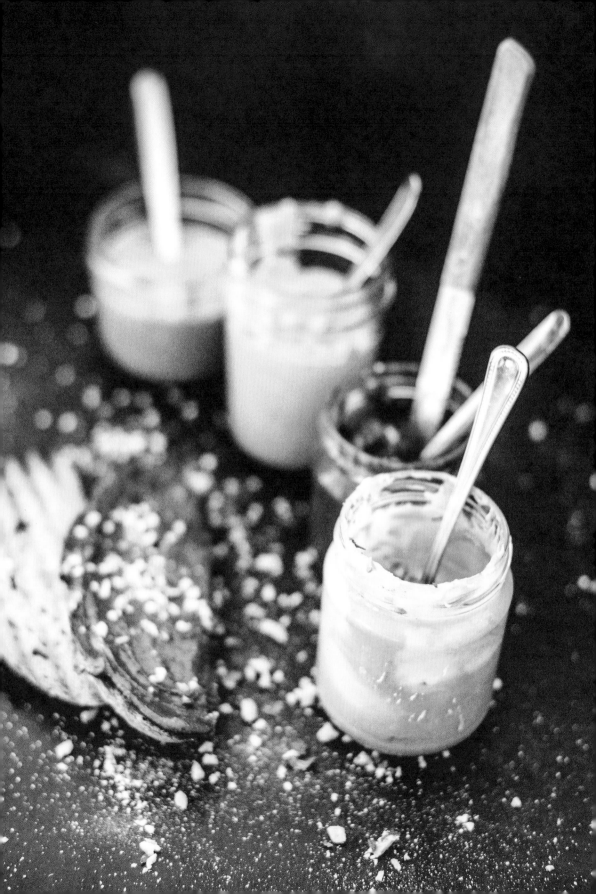

Milk Varieties

When it comes to the choice of which milk to use for each recipe, you're pretty free – just like in the choice of which natural sweetener to use. The types of milk I use most often are unsweetened soy, rice and almond milk. Other options are oat, spelt and other nut milks. If you use cow's milk, I recommend skimmed (low-fat) milk.

Whatever milk you buy, always make sure you buy unsweetened varieties because some may contain refined sugar. If you're new to non-dairy plant alternatives, you should definitely buy a variety of different types so that you can find out what your preference is.

SOY MILK
(43 CAL/180 KJ PER 100 ML/3½ FL OZ)
Soy milk is the variety of milk I use most often. It is made of dried, ground soybeans with the addition of water and is suitable if you're intolerant to lactose and/or gluten. It's a purely plant-based product and a good source of vitamins, calcium and potassium. Soy milk can, depending on the brand, almost contain as much calcium as cow's milk and tastes incredibly delicious sweetened with some coconut nectar.

RICE MILK
(50 CAL/209 KJ PER 100 ML/3½ FL OZ)
Rice milk is lovely because of its naturally sweet taste. I love to drink a glass of cool rice milk in between meals, not only to satisfy my thirst but also when I'm craving something sweet. Rice milk is produced from ground rice with the addition of water. It's also suitable for people intolerant to nuts, lactose and gluten. Rice milk is rich in carbohydrates and contains little protein compared to other types of milk.

ALMOND MILK
(42 CAL/176 KJ PER 100 ML/3½ FL OZ)
Almond milk is slightly thicker than other types of milk. You should always shake the milk well before using it so that the tiny almond-particles are mixed up with the liquid. Otherwise, the almond pieces separate from the liquid and settle at the bottom. Almond milk has a nutty flavour and can be used for a range of dishes. I often use it for my breakfast or in my healthy dessert recipes. It provides plenty of the valuable vitamins A and D, and it's also free from lactose.

OAT MILK
(40 CAL/167 KJ PER 100 ML/3½ FL OZ)
Oat milk naturally has a slightly sweet and nutty flavour. It's also a great kind of milk to use for cooking, baking and to use in breakfast recipes. The plant-based milk is produced from fermented oats and water. It contains gluten, but no lactose. Oat milk is rich in minerals and vitamins, has a low fat content and is easy to digest.

SKIMMED MILK
(47 CAL/197 KJ PER 100 ML/3½ FL OZ)
Normal cow's milk has a fat content of 3.5 percent, skimmed has a fat content of only 0.1 percent and is therefore accordingly low in calories. Cow's milk with a fat content of more than 0.5 percent is called low-fat milk and no longer skimmed milk. Cow's milk is probably the cheapest kind of milk on the market. It contains lactose and is not suitable for vegans.

COCONUT MILK
(33 CAL/824 KJ PER 100 ML/3½ FL OZ)
See page 29.

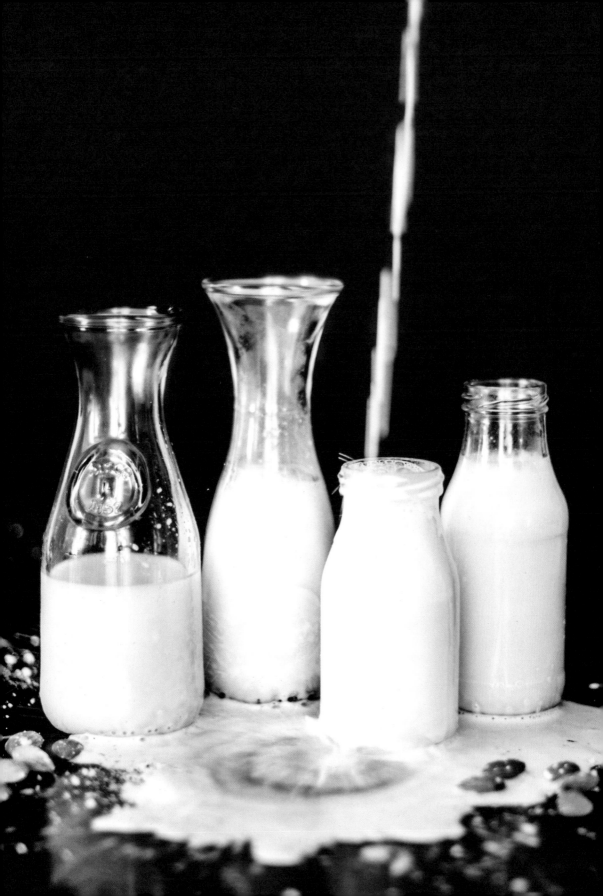

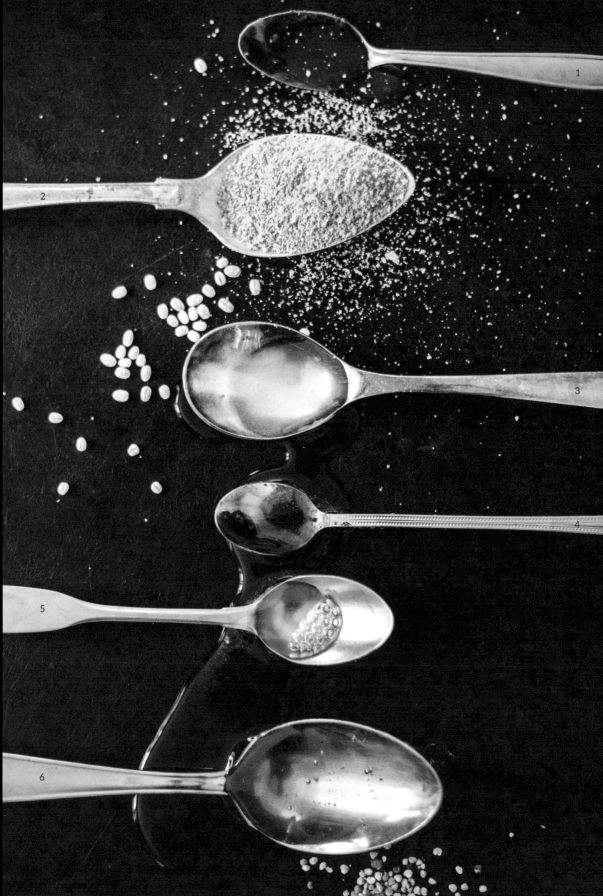

Sweeteners

Something that is really important to me and is a big part of the philosophy behind *Eat Better Not Less* is not eating white, refined sugar. It has, almost exclusively, negative effects on the body; it makes you tired and sluggish, robs your energy and increases your desire for sweets. Refined sugar is hidden in an incredible array of foods, many of which you would never think of. Therefore, I advise to always double-check if the products you're buying contain any refined sugar. The human body needs sugar, but natural sugar. The sugar in fruit, vegetables, plant-based and wholesome products is necessary. There are plenty of good and natural alternatives to refined sugar. Some are more neutral in their taste while others have a stronger, more unique taste. In my recipes, you can select the sweetener you prefer. Of course, the flavour can vary depending on what you choose for each recipe. However, that doesn't matter as a variety of flavours can make the dish more interesting. Whichever sweetener you choose, make sure to buy the 100 percent pure and natural version.

All of these natural sweeteners contain simple sugar in the form of fructose and should therefore be enjoyed in moderation. I personally love to add a teaspoon or two to my dishes, sweet or savoury. For me, taste comes first. I can't enjoy eating something I don't like and which leaves me thinking it would be better if it were a bit sweeter. However, everyone has a different preference for sweetness. You can decide for yourself whether you want to use a little more or less sweetener in your food.

HONEY
(21 CAL/88 KJ PER TEASPOON)

I use honey most often to sweeten my breakfasts or for salad dressings. Compared to agave nectar, honey has a stronger, sweeter taste. It contains vitamins and minerals and doesn't increase blood sugar levels as fast as other sweeteners.

AGAVE NECTAR
(20 CAL/84 KJ PER TEASPOON)

The taste and consistency of agave nectar can be compared to that of honey. Thanks to its natural taste, it can be used for almost any kind of dish. Amongst the listed sweeteners, agave nectar has the highest amount of fructose.

MAPLE SYRUP
(17 CAL/71 KJ PER TEASPOON)

Maple syrup is another ideal sweetener for salad dressings or my healthy dessert recipes. I find maple syrup fairly sweet and like to use it for baking. Make sure to buy pure, natural maple syrup without any added sugar.

RICE SYRUP / BROWN RICE SYRUP
(25 CAL/105 KJ PER TEASPOON)

Rice syrup is one of my absolute favourite sweeteners for breakfasts, shakes, smoothies and desserts. It has a slightly thicker consistency than honey. It's best to use brown rice syrup, but if you can't find it, you can also use regular white rice syrup.

COCONUT SUGAR
(15 CAL/63 KJ PER TEASPOON)

Coconut sugar is made from coconut flower buds. It contains a lot of minerals and vitamins. Although it's not the sweetest, it's incredibly tasty. It's great to sprinkle on top of smoothies or any kind of breakfast. Not only does it look fantastic, it also brings a delicious caramel note to any dish.

COCONUT NECTAR
(18 CAL/75 KJ PER TEASPOON)

The liquid, almost sticky coconut nectar is the raw by-product of coconut blossom sugar. It has quite a strong taste. If you like it, coconut nectar can be used for a wide variety of dishes, although I mainly recommend it for breakfast and dessert recipes.

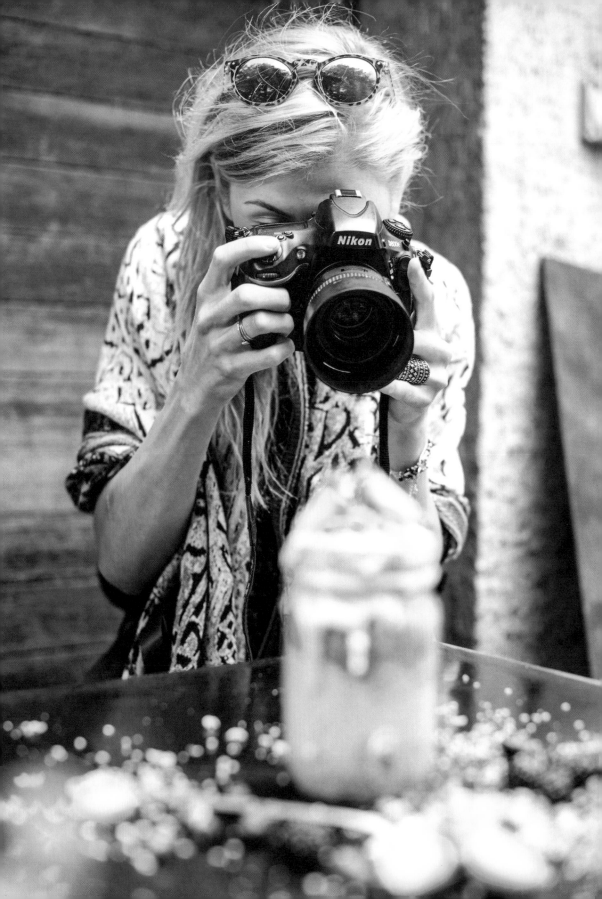

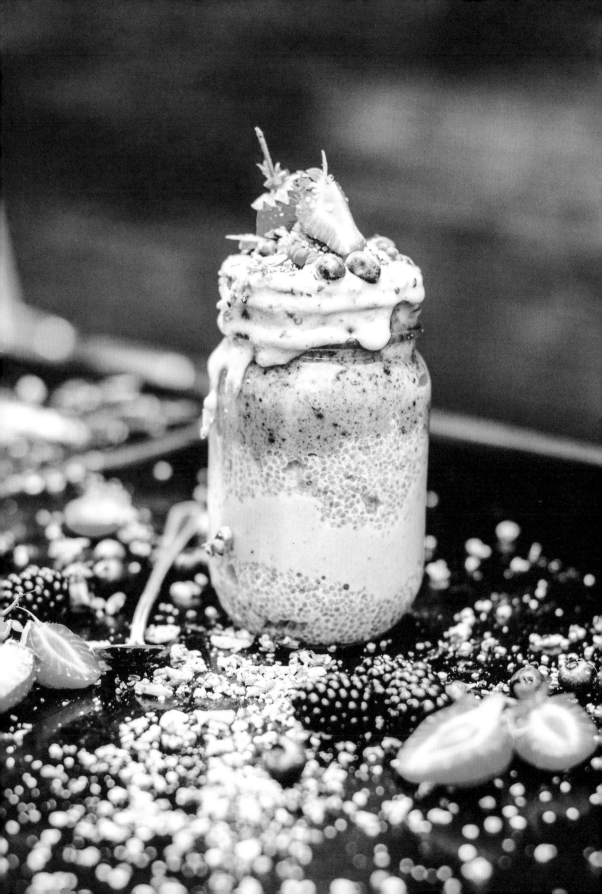

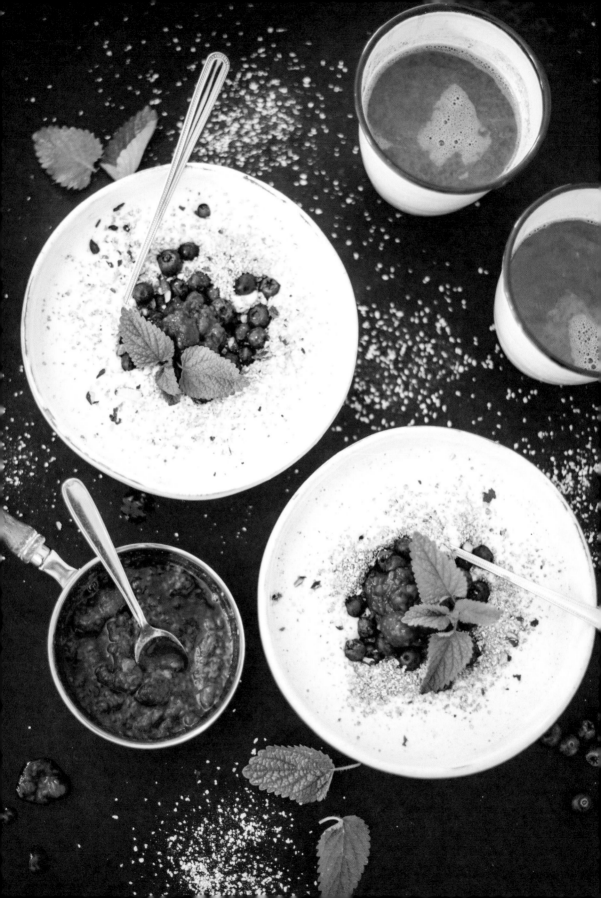

BREAKFAST

How to start the day off right

GF= GLUTEN-FREE · DF= DAIRY-FREE
V= VEGETARIAN · VGN= VEGAN · RSF= REFINED-SUGAR-FREE

Dreamy Cashew & Banana Ice Cream with Strawberry Coulis

This combination will make your heart melt!

Something I just can't resist is banana ice cream for breakfast. You're probably thinking, 'What?! Ice cream for breakfast?' Yes, that's right: ice cream for breakfast. And not just any kind of ice cream; it's the best and healthiest ice cream there is and it's very easy to make. All you have to do in advance is peel some ripe bananas, cut them into slices and freeze them overnight. A good blender or food processor is highly recommended for a creamy and smooth result. You haven't tried it yet? Then it's about time you do. I promise you, if you like bananas, you will absolutely love banana ice cream.

—————————— SERVES 1 / GF, DF, VGN, RSF ——————————

BANANA ICE CREAM

2 bananas, sliced and frozen

100 ml (3½ fl oz) milk of choice, e.g. soy, almond, rice milk

1–2 teaspoons maple syrup or sweetener of choice (optional)

10–14 cashews or 1 tablespoon cashew butter

2 dates, pitted

8 strawberries, diced

STRAWBERRY-COULIS

8 strawberries

few drops of vanilla extract

1–2 teaspoons maple syrup or sweetener of choice

2 tablespoons water

crushed cashews, to garnish

1   To make the ice cream, remove the frozen banana slices from the freezer and let them thaw for a few minutes. Put them into a blender or food processor together with the milk, maple syrup (if using), cashews and dates, then blend until smooth and creamy.

2   For the coulis, cut the strawberries into small pieces. Cook them in a small saucepan over a medium heat together with the vanilla extract, maple syrup and water for about 4–5 minutes. Take off the heat and let it cool.

3   Layer the banana ice cream and fresh strawberries alternately into a jar, finishing with the banana ice cream. Top with the strawberry coulis and sprinkle some crushed cashews on top. Enjoy right away.

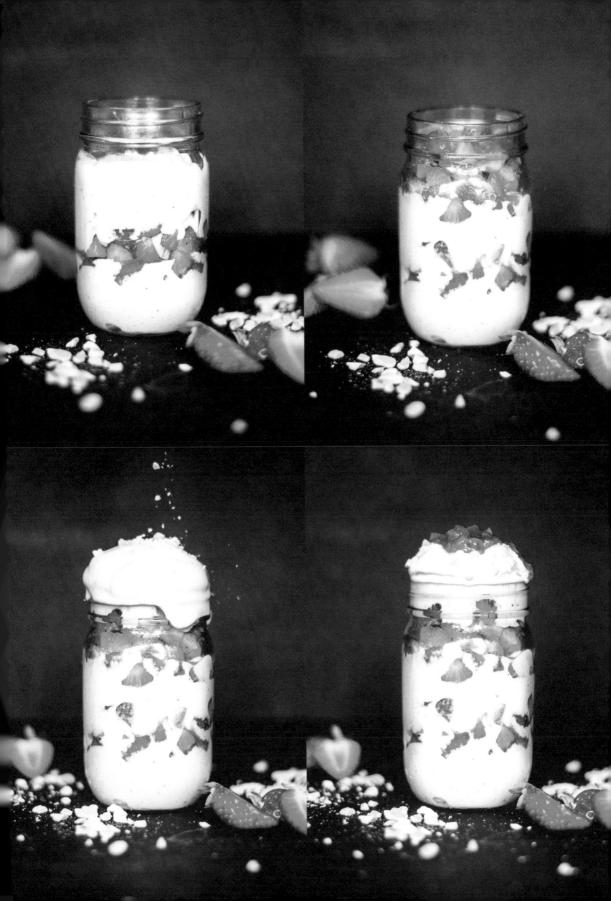

Blueberry & Almond Bowl

An ice-cold superfood breakfast to get you energised.
This bowl is so refreshing, fruity and easy to make. The almond extract and cinnamon gives it such a delicious taste that you definitely shouldn't miss out on. The almond butter makes this ice-cold smoothie so creamy and the spinach provides extra iron without changing the taste. Topped with chia seeds, fresh blueberries, toasted almonds and sunflower seeds, this is a perfect combination.

SERVES 1 / GF, DF, VGN, RSF

BLUEBERRY CREAM

250 g (9 oz) frozen blueberries

1 banana

200 ml (7 fl oz) almond milk or nut milk of choice

2 teaspoons maple syrup or sweetener of choice

1 teaspoon chia seeds

1 teaspoon sunflower seeds

few drops of bitter almond extract

2–3 teaspoons almond butter

1 teaspoon cinnamon

2 handfuls spinach

TOPPINGS

1 tablespoon flaked (slivered) almonds

2 teaspoon sunflower seeds

1 teaspoon chia seeds

1–2 tablespoons fresh or frozen and thawed blueberries

1   For the blueberry cream, use a food processor to blend all the ingredients to a smooth and creamy consistency, until none of the spinach leaves are visible. Pour into a bowl.

2   Toast the flaked almonds in a dry frying pan (skillet) over a medium heat until golden brown. Take off the heat and let them cool.

3   Top the blueberry cream with the toasted almonds, sunflower seeds, chia seeds and blueberries.

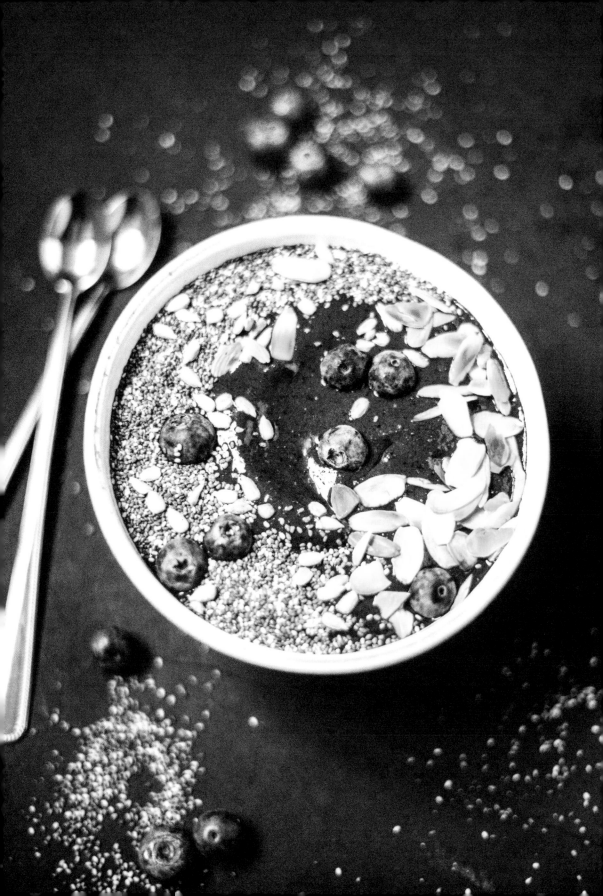

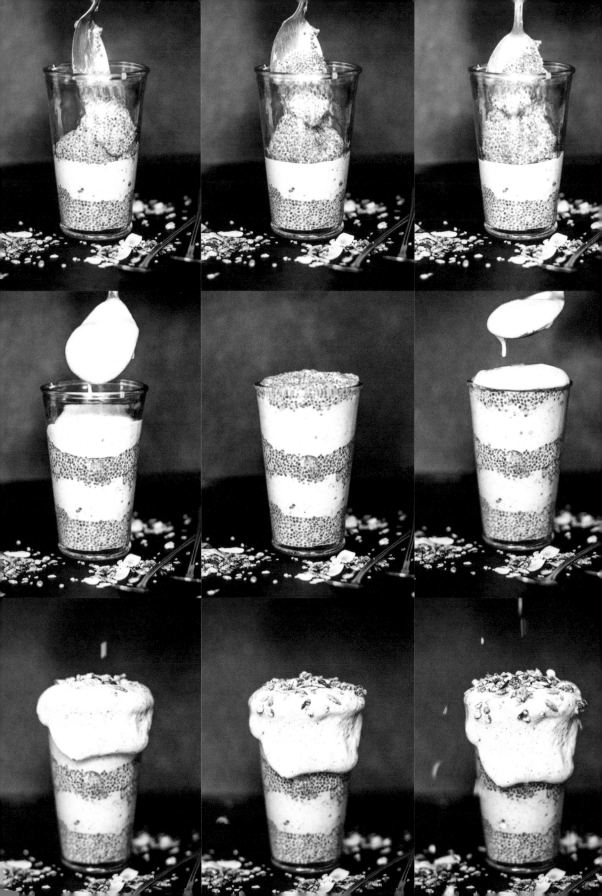

Carob & Banana Ice Cream with Vanilla Chia Pudding

A breakfast to enjoy layer by layer.

It's no secret any more that I'm absolutely crazy about banana ice cream. I've recently started to fall in love with chia pudding as well. Instead of choosing between banana ice cream and chia pudding, I simply decided to combine them in one breakfast. Even though the textures and tastes are completely different, they go so well together. If you have not come across carob powder yet you should definitely give it a try! It's an alternative to cacao powder and has a pretty strong, delicious taste. It is best to prepare the chia pudding the night before because the seeds need to soak to achieve a thick consistency.

-------- SERVES 1-2 / GF, DF, VGN, RSF --------

CHIA PUDDING

3 tablespoons chia seeds

300 ml (10½ fl oz) milk of choice, e.g. soy, almond, rice milk

1 teaspoon vanilla extract

2–3 teaspoons maple syrup or sweetener of choice

BANANA ICE CREAM

2 bananas, sliced and frozen

100 ml (3½ fl oz) milk of choice, e.g. soy, almond, rice milk

1 tablespoon carob powder

2 dates, pitted and cut into smaller pieces

1–2 teaspoons maple syrup or sweetener of choice

crushed nuts of choice, to serve

1–2 teaspoon chia seeds, to serve

1   To make the chia pudding, add the chia seeds, milk, vanilla extract and maple syrup into a bowl and stir until well combined. Soak in the fridge overnight or for at least 2 hours.

2   For the banana ice cream, take the frozen banana slices out of the freezer. Leave to thaw for a few minutes, then put them into a blender or food processor together with the milk. Blend until smooth and creamy. Add the carob powder, dates and maple syrup and mix for another minute.

3   Stir the chia pudding again to break up any lumps. and layer into a jar, alternating with the banana ice cream. Sprinkle some crushed nuts and chia seeds on top and enjoy.

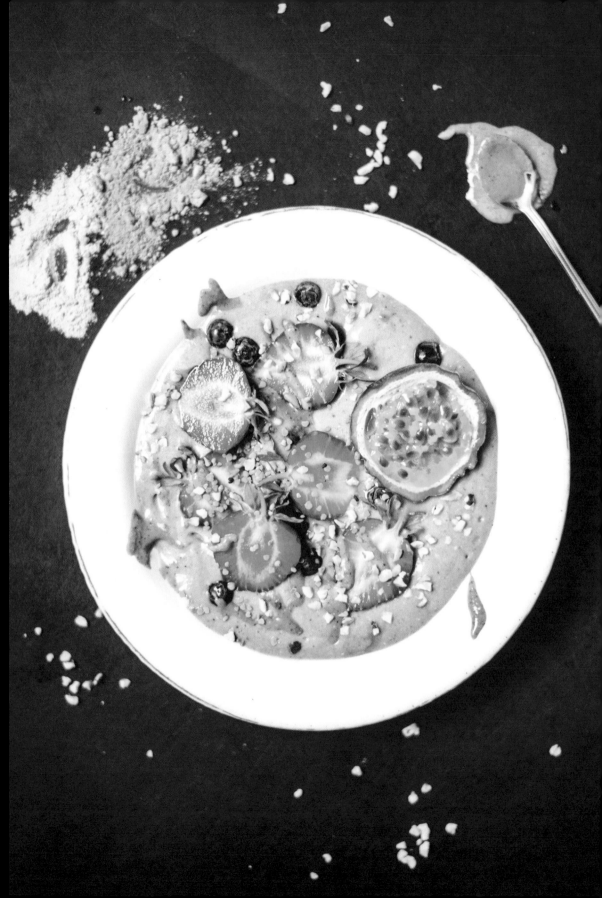

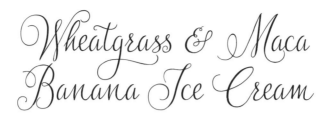

Wheatgrass & Maca Banana Ice Cream

A green wonder topped with lots of goodies.

Wheatgrass and maca powder are two of my favourite superfoods to add to my breakfast. Not only do they provide plenty of energy, they also taste really good when added to banana ice cream, porridge (oatmeal), shakes and smoothies. You can get them at pretty much every health food store or order them online. The pistachio and coconut butter used in this recipe is home-made (recipe on page 36). Topping this breakfast bowl with fresh fruit and some crushed nuts guarantees a good start to a new day.

SERVES 1 / GF, DF, VGN, RSF

BANANA ICE CREAM

2 bananas, sliced and frozen

150 ml (5 fl oz) milk of choice, e.g. soy, almond, rice milk

1–2 teaspoons wheatgrass powder

1–2 teaspoons maca powder

few drops of vanilla extract

2–3 teaspoons maple syrup or sweetener of choice

2 teaspoons Pistachio & Coconut Butter (see page 36) or almond butter

TOPPINGS

fruit of choice, e.g. strawberries, blueberries, passion fruit

crushed nuts of choice

2 teaspoons Pistachio & Coconut Butter (see page 36) or almond butter

1   Take the frozen banana slices out of the freezer and allow them to thaw for a few minutes. Put them into a blender or food processor together with the milk and blend until smooth and creamy.

2   Add the remaining ingredients for the ice cream and blend for another minute until well combined.

3   Pour into a bowl, top with your fruit of choice and the crushed nuts and drizzle some pistachio and coconut butter on top.

WHEATGRASS   Contains over 60 times more vitamin C than oranges, is good for the digestion and is alkalising, helping to balance the body's pH levels. In addition, it provides a lot of energy and fights tiredness. A real superfood, I'd say!

My Kind of Acai Bowl

Bursts of colour, fresh ingredients and a fusion of flavours can only taste good.
If you ever get up on the wrong side of the bed, this breakfast will save your day.
I absolutely love having an acai bowl with as many of my favourite toppings as possible
for breakfast. The acai berry, from South America, not only has an irresistible taste,
it's also rich in antioxidants. Since the fresh berries are not available here in Switzerland,
I use the acai powder. The powder can be quite expensive, but it's so worth it.
I wanted to create my very own acai bowl recipe and this one had me hooked from the
very first mouthful. Try it for yourself!

————————— SERVES 1 / GF, DF, VGN, RSF —————————

ACAI BOWL

1 banana, sliced and frozen

150 g (5 oz) frozen blackberries
   or blueberries

2 tablespoons acai powder

½ apple

2 teaspoons maple syrup or sweetener
   of choice

2 teaspoons almond butter

100 ml (3½ fl oz) almond milk or milk
   of choice

100 ml (3½ fl oz) coconut water

TOPPING IDEAS

berries of choice, e.g. strawberries,
   raspberries, blueberries

dried mulberries

bee pollen

unsweetened coconut chips

Crunchy Cinnamon Granola (see page 104)

roasted nuts of choice

sliced banana

1   Put all of the acai bowl ingredients into a blender or food processor and blend for a few minutes until smooth and creamy.

2   Pour into a bowl and sprinkle with your favourite toppings. I love adding some granola, home-made coconut chips and/or roasted nuts to give it some extra crunchiness.

3   Enjoy every single spoonful – the bowl will be empty faster than you would like!

VARIATION   Use 200 ml (7 fl oz) of almond milk or coconut water instead of a mixture of the two.

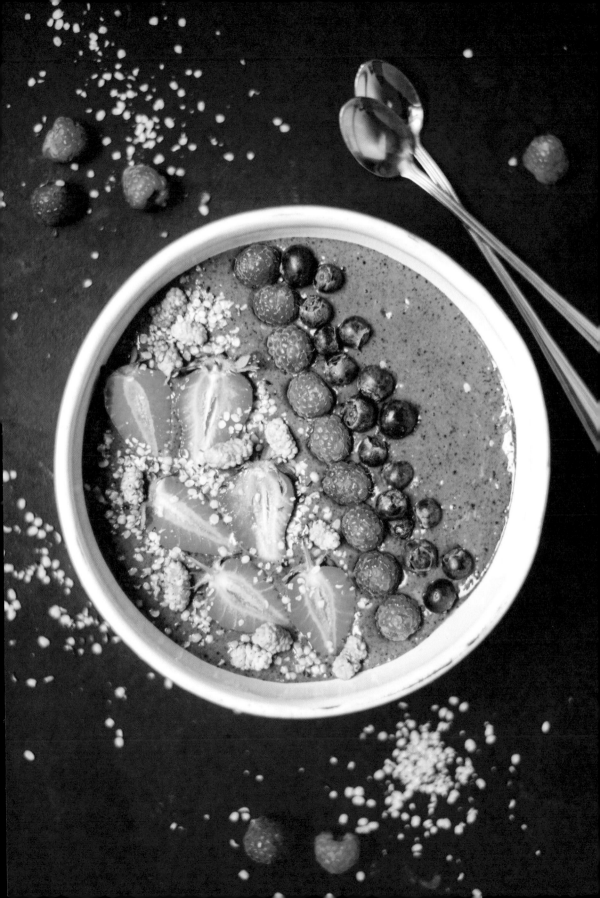

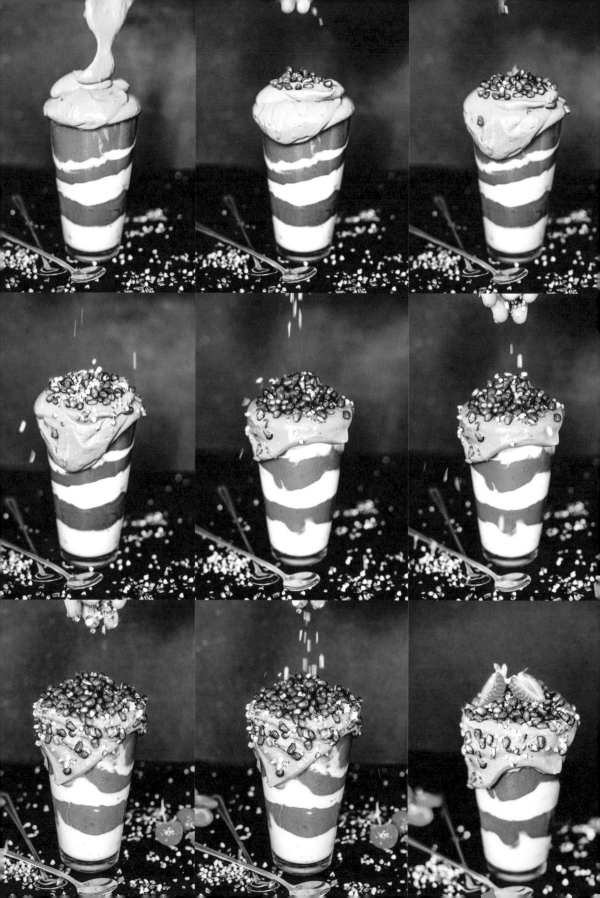

Vanilla, Cacao & Peanut Banana Ice Cream

When a breakfast turns into a dessert, or the other way around.
Looking at this picture you're probably thinking it's a dessert full of chocolate, cream and sugar. That's not the case, though; this recipe is dairy-free and doesn't contain any additives. This jar of deliciousness only contains natural ingredients and therefore can be enjoyed completely guilt-free. This is definitely one of my favourite variations of banana ice cream because it contains three of my favourite ingredients: banana, cacao and home-made peanut butter. For those who love to have something sweet for breakfast, this recipe is made for you. This can also be served for dessert in smaller portions.

SERVES 1-2 / GF, DF, VGN, RSF

VANILLA BANANA ICE CREAM

1–1½ bananas, sliced and frozen

1 vanilla bean, seeds scraped

100 ml (3½ fl oz) milk of choice, e.g. soy, almond, rice milk

1–2 teaspoons maple syrup or sweetener of choice

CACAO & PEANUT BANANA ICE CREAM

1–1½ bananas, sliced and frozen

100 ml (3½ fl oz) milk of choice, e.g. soy, almond, rice milk

1 teaspoon cacao powder

1 tablespoon peanut butter

1–2 teaspoons maple syrup or sweetener of choice

TOPPINGS

pomegranate seeds

berries of choice

2–3 teaspoons cacao nibs

crushed nuts of choice

1   For the vanilla banana ice cream, take the frozen banana slices out of the freezer. Leave to thaw for a few minutes.

2   Put all the ingredients for the vanilla ice cream into a blender or food processor and blend for a few minutes until smooth and creamy. Repeat for the cacao and peanut ice cream, remembering to allow the bananas to thaw first.

3   Fill a jar layer by layer, alternating between the two different kinds of banana ice cream.

4   Top with pomegranate seeds and berries and, for some crunch, sprinkle over some cacao nibs and crushed nuts.

PEANUT BUTTER   If you buy ready-made peanut butter, make sure to buy the version without added sugar or oils.

Blueberry Quinoa with Banana Ice Cream & Berries

A summer dream come true.

I absolutely love this breakfast! Having this jar in front of me gets me into a good mood instantly. If the banana ice cream has the right consistency, it stays firm and doesn't run over the sides of the glass. To achieve this effect, it's important to thaw the frozen banana slices for a few minutes so that you don't have to add too much liquid when blending. The combination of the creamy blueberry quinoa and fresh berries is simply to die for. A breakfast that will fill you up with sunshine and keep you satisfied for a few hours.

SERVES 3-4 / GF, DF, VGN, RSF

QUINOA

2–3 tablespoons quinoa

100 ml (3½ fl oz) water

pinch of salt

100 ml (3½ fl oz) milk of choice, e.g. soy, almond, rice milk

1 teaspoon maple syrup or sweetener of choice

3 tablespoons frozen blueberries

BANANA ICE CREAM

2 bananas, sliced and frozen

100 ml (3½ fl oz) milk of choice, e.g. soy, almond, rice milk

few drops of pure vanilla extract

2–3 teaspoons maple syrup or sweetener of choice

2 handfuls of fresh berries of choice

crushed nuts of choice

1   Start by making the quinoa. Put the water and salt into a saucepan over a high heat and bring to the boil. Turn down the heat to medium, add the remaining ingredients, stir well and let it cook for 9–12 minutes until the quinoa is tender. Add another splash of milk if desired.

2   Meanwhile, take the frozen banana slices out of the freezer and thaw for a few minutes. Put them into a blender or food processor together with the milk, vanilla extract and maple syrup, and blend until smooth and creamy.

3   Spoon half of the banana ice cream into a jar, add the fresh berries on top, followed by the cooked blueberry quinoa, the rest of the berries and then the remaining banana ice cream.

4   Sprinkle some crushed nuts on top and enjoy.

TIP   Use a long spoon to eat this breakfast and dive right to the bottom. By doing so you will get the full taste experience of all the different layers combined.

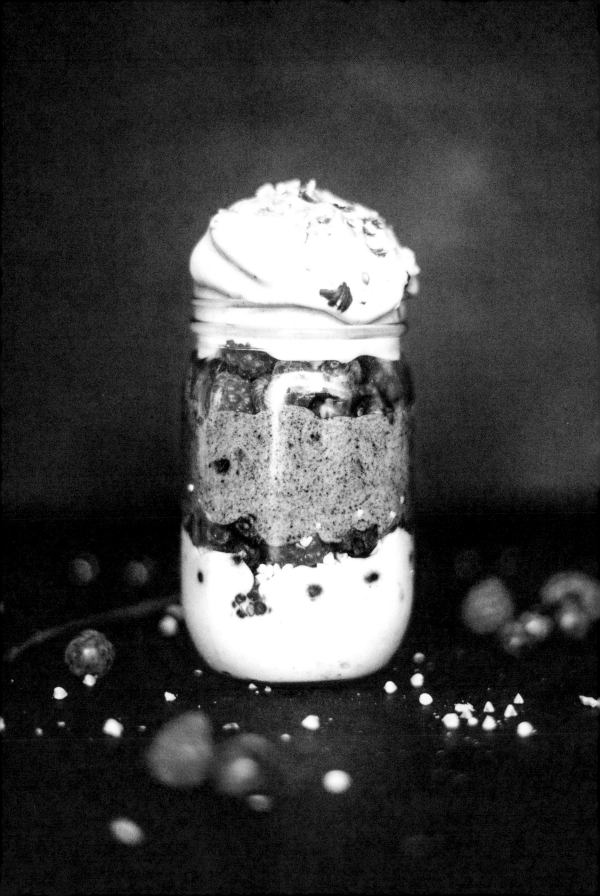

Ovaltine Banana Ice Cream

The real Swiss deal!

Back in the day I drank an Ovomaltine – called Ovaltine outside of Switzerland – almost every day. In summer I had it with cold milk and in winter with hot milk. Ovomaltine contains barley malt, and many vitamins and minerals. The original version also contains sugar, but a sugar-free version is available in Switzerland. If you can't find this, it can be substitued with Ovaltine Light. Since I like adding raw cacao powder to banana ice cream, the idea of adding Ovomaltine with its slightly more chocolatey taste came to my mind. I enjoyed every single spoonful and had flashbacks to my childhood.

SERVES 1 / RSF

BANANA ICE CREAM

2–3 bananas, frozen and sliced

150 ml (5 fl oz) milk of choice, e.g. soy, almond, rice milk

few drops of pure vanilla extract

2–3 tablespoons sugar-free Ovomaltine or Ovaltine Light

2 teaspoons maple syrup or sweetener of choice

2 teaspoons peanut butter

TOPPINGS

cacao nibs

berries of choice

crushed nuts of choice, e.g. peanuts, almonds, cashews

1   Take the frozen banana slices out of the freezer and thaw for a few minutes.

2   Put the bananas into the blender or food processor with the remaining ingredients for the ice cream and blend until smooth and creamy.

3   Pour into a bowl or deep plate and top with cacao nibs, berries and crushed nuts.

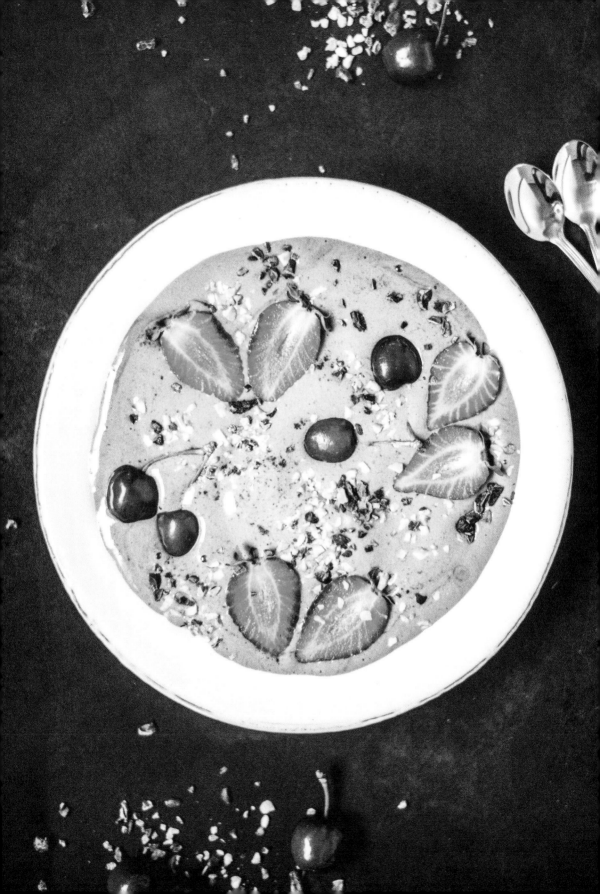

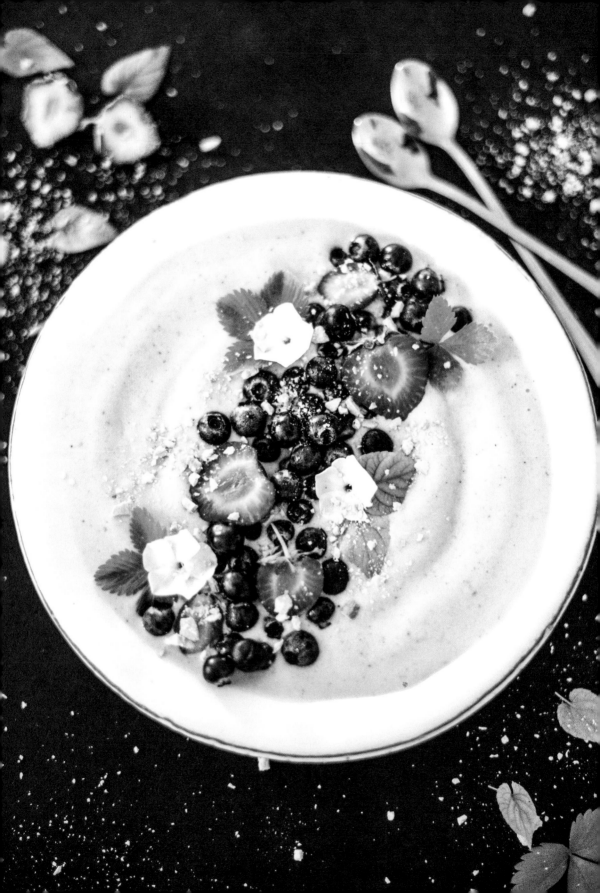

Maca & Peanut Banana Ice Cream

A dream-team combination and almost too good to eat.
I can't get enough of banana ice cream. The good thing about it, though, is that it never gets boring because you can make an infinite number of variations. Maca powder, derived from the maca root, has such a great taste. It also has many health benefits: it's rich in vitamins and not only provides you with energy but also strengthens your mind and improves concentration. If you're not yet familiar with maca, you should run to the nearest health food store and get it. Together with the peanut butter it simply tastes AH-MAZING!

SERVES 1 / GF, DF, VGN, RSF

BANANA ICE CREAM

2 bananas, sliced and frozen

150 ml (5 fl oz) milk of choice, e.g. soy, almond, rice milk

1 tablespoon peanut butter

2 teaspoons maca powder

1 vanilla bean, seeds scraped

2 teaspoons maple syrup or sweetener of choice

TOPPINGS

berries or fruit of choice

crushed peanuts

hemp seeds

1 Take the frozen banana slices out of the freezer and leave to thaw for a few minutes. Put them into a blender or food processor with all the other ice cream ingredients and blend until smooth and creamy.

2 Spoon the banana ice cream into a deep dish and top with the fruit, crushed peanuts and hemp seeds.

TO ALL THE PEANUT LOVERS   Sometimes less is more and sometimes more is more. In this case, more is more. Use a fork to mix 1–2 teaspoons of peanut butter in a small bowl with a splash of milk until smooth. Drizzle on top of the banana ice cream.

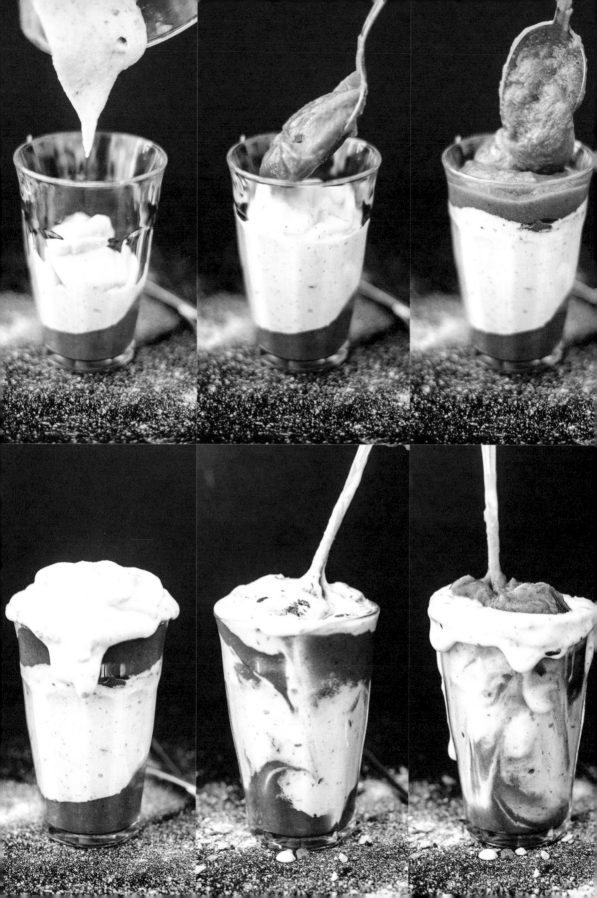

Banana Ice Cream with a Date Caramel Swirl

For those who like it extra sweet.

Don't we all have a weakness for sweet things like chocolate, caramel and desserts in general? I think once in a while everyone craves something sweet! This recipe is so simple and all you need are five ingredients. The sweet Medjool dates taste so similar to caramel you won't even miss it a bit. I love to eat this for breakfast because I need something sweet in the morning. However, it's great to serve as a dessert if you don't fancy something sweet for breakfast.

SERVES 1 / GF, DF, VGN, RSF

BANANA ICE CREAM

2 bananas, sliced and frozen

splash of milk of choice, e.g. soy, almond, rice milk

few drops of vanilla extract

DATE CARAMEL

4 Mejdool dates, pitted

100 ml (3½ fl oz) water

1   Take the frozen banana slices out of the freezer and leave to thaw for a few minutes.

2   In the meantime, make the caramel. Blend the Medjool dates together with the water until it reaches a smooth consistency. You might have to add another splash of water depending on the size of the dates. Put the banana slices together with the milk and vanilla extract into a blender or food processor and blend until smooth and creamy.

3   Put the banana slices together with the milk and vanilla extract into a blender or food processor and blend until smooth and creamy.

4   Spoon half of the date caramel into a jar. Pour in the banana ice cream, top with the rest of the date caramel and give it a quick stir to create a swirl. Don't mix completely: left like this every spoonful tastes a bit different and makes eating this jar of sweet deliciousness even more exciting.

DATES   If you don't have Medjool dates, use about 6 smaller dates instead. Boil them until soft, then drain and blend them with water until smooth.

Coconut Banana Ice Cream with Three-Ingredient Chocolate Sauce

Coconut lovers get blending – this one's for you!

Some people don't like it, some love it and some are crazy about it. I belong to group number three and love everything coconut. The chocolate sauce in this recipe is made in just a few minutes and contains only three ingredients. Since the banana ice cream is frozen and the chocolate sauce is hot, it sets immediately when drizzled over the ice cream and tastes just like chocolate. You can get coconut nectar at almost every health food store. It has a stronger taste than other sweeteners and has a slightly sticky consistency, but it goes so well with this recipe and brings out the coconut flavour even more.

———————————— SERVES 1 / GF, DF, VGN, RSF ————————————

BANANA ICE CREAM

2 bananas, sliced and frozen

1 tablespoon coconut butter or 2 tablespoons shredded coconut

150 ml (5 fl oz) coconut milk

2–3 teaspoons maple syrup or sweetener of choice

CHOCOLATE SAUCE

1 tablespoon coconut oil

1 tablespoon raw cacao powder

1 tablespoon coconut nectar

TOPPINGS

fresh or frozen and thawed berries of choice

Sesame Coconut Chips (see page 96)

1   Take the frozen banana slices out of the freezer and leave to thaw for a few minutes.

2   In the meantime, make the chocolate sauce. In a small saucepan heat up the coconut oil until it becomes liquid. Add the raw cacao powder and coconut nectar, stir well, and leave on the stove but turn off the heat.

3   To make the ice cream, put the banana slices into a blender together with the coconut butter, milk and sweetener and blend to a smooth and creamy consistency.

4   Pour the ice cream into a bowl (I used a hollow coconut shell) and drizzle the warm chocolate sauce on top.

5   Top with berries and coconut chips and experience coconut heaven!

VARIATIONS   If you don't have any coconut nectar on hand, you can also use other sweeteners for the chocolate sauce such as honey or maple syrup. The ratio for the chocolate sauce ingredients is always 1:1:1.

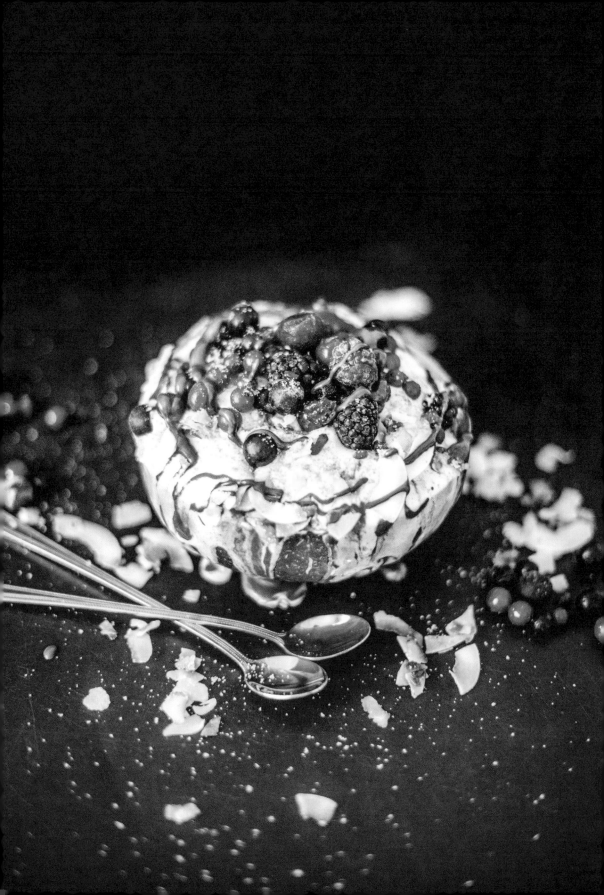

Cacao & Banana Porridge

A sweet temptation for breakfast.

This porridge will make every chocolate lover's heart beat faster. But can something this chocolatey for breakfast actually be healthy? Yes, of course it can! Anyone who claims that you have to say no to the taste of chocolate in a balanced diet is wrong. The secret ingredient is called raw cacao powder (see page 29) and, combined with natural sweeteners or sweet fruit like banana, creates the chocolate taste you're looking for. Adding some peanut butter turns this bowl into a breakfast everybody will love.

——————————— SERVES 1 / (GF), DF, VGN, RSF ———————————

PORRIDGE (OATMEAL)

200 ml (7 fl oz) water

pinch of salt

4–5 tablespoons porridge oats (oatmeal) (gluten-free)

1 ripe banana

200 ml (7 fl oz) milk of choice, e.g. soy, almond, rice milk

2 teaspoons peanut butter

2 teaspoons maple syrup or sweetener of choice

2 tablespoons raw cacao powder

CHOCOLATE SAUCE

2 teaspoons water

1 teaspoons coconut oil, melted

2 teaspoons raw cacao powder

1–2 teaspoons maple syrup or sweetener of choice

TOPPINGS

½ banana, sliced

blueberries

crushed nuts of choice

1   First, make the porridge. In a saucepan, bring the water to the boil, add the salt and oats, and cook for 2–3 minutes. Meanwhile, mash the banana with a fork.

2   Turn down the heat, then add the mashed banana along with the milk, peanut butter, maple syrup and cacao powder. Stir well and let it cook for about 4–5 minutes. Stir from time to time.

3   For the chocolate sauce, mix all the ingredients in a small jar until smooth.

4   Add another splash of milk to the porridge if desired, take off the heat and pour into a bowl.

5   Top with fresh banana slices, blueberries and, of course, the chocolate sauce. Finish off with some crushed nuts.

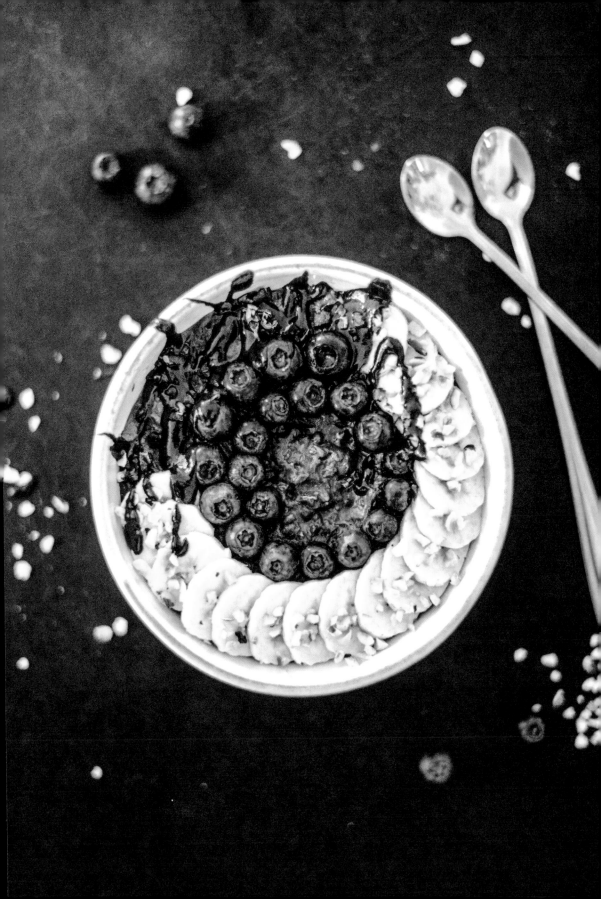

Creamy Vanilla Quinoa Porridge with Berries

Quinoa: also great in sweet dishes.

Most of you probably know quinoa made with vegetables and in savoury dishes. But sweet quinoa is just as good, if not better. To sweeten, I love using natural ingredients – sometimes a ripe banana is all it needs. You can enjoy this bowl right away or cool it in the fridge and enjoy it the next morning, or even bring it with you for lunch. I love eating this porridge (oatmeal) once it has cooled for a few hours in the fridge because the flavours are enhanced. It's also a great breakfast to prepare the night before if you don't have time in the morning. I'd recommend only adding the fruit and nuts just before eating.

—————————— SERVES 1 / GF, DF, VGN, RSF ——————————

PORRIDGE (OATMEAL)

150 ml (5 fl oz) water

pinch of salt

3–4 tablespoons quinoa

250 ml (8½ fl oz) milk of choice, e.g. soy, almond, rice milk

1 ripe banana

1 tablespoon peanut butter

2–3 teaspoons maple syrup or sweetener of choice

1 vanilla bean, seeds scraped

TOPPINGS

raspberries

strawberries

pomegranate seeds

crushed nuts of choice, roasted (optional)

1   Bring the water and salt to the boil in a saucepan. Add the quinoa, turn down the heat slightly, then add 150 ml (5 fl oz) of the milk and cook for 6–8 minutes.

2   Mash the banana with a fork and add to the quinoa. Then stir in the peanut butter, maple syrup and vanilla seeds, and cook for a few more minutes.

3   Take off the heat, add the remaining milk and stir well.

4   Pour the porridge into a bowl. Top with the berries, pomegranate seeds and for the perfect crunch, sprinkle crushed (and preferably roasted) nuts on top.

VARIATIONS   You can also use frozen berries and thaw them before adding them on top of the porridge. If you don't like berries, mango, passion fruit or other tropical fruit also go well with this quinoa porridge.

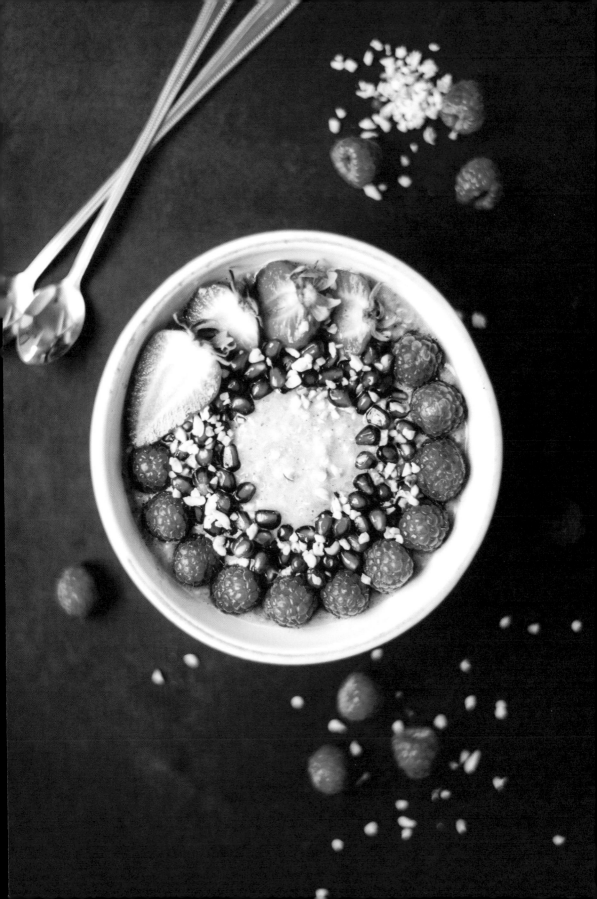

Four Kinds of Fruity Oats

Same, same but different.

It's always a great idea to start the day off with an energising, filling, nutritious and delicious bowl of porridge. Apart from that, it literally only takes you five minutes to make and there are so many different ways to pimp up your oats. Here are four easy fruit and nut porridge creations for you to choose from. You can even come up with your very own combinations. Set your taste buds and creativity to ON and you'll be the next oat chef in no time! Oh, and for the best flavour, make sure to only use roasted nuts.

FOR 1 PORTION EACH / (GF), DF, VGN, RSF

PORRIDGE (OATMEAL)

100 ml (3½ fl oz) water

pinch of salt

4 tablespoons oats (oatmeal) (gluten-free)

150 ml (5 fl oz) milk of choice, e.g. soy, almond, rice milk

1 small ripe banana

1–2 teaspoons maple syrup or sweetener of choice

few drops of vanilla extract

STRAWBERRY & HAZELNUT

6–8 strawberries, plus extra to serve

1 teaspoon maple syrup or sweetener of choice

1 tablespoon water

1 tablespoon hazelnuts, roasted and crushed, or 1 tablespoon hazelnut butter, to serve

RASPBERRY & CASHEW

2–4 tablespoons raspberries, plus extra to serve

1 teaspoon maple syrup or sweetener of choice

1 tablespoon water

1 tablespoon cashews, roasted and crushed, or 1 tablespoon cashew butter, to serve

BLUEBERRY & PISTACHIO

2–3 tablespoons blueberries, plus extra to serve

1 teaspoon maple syrup or sweetener of choice

1 tablespoon water

1 tablespoon pistachios, roasted and crushed, or 1 tablespoon pistachio butter, to serve

POMEGRANATE & PECAN

2–3 tablespoons pomegranate seeds, plus extra to serve

1 teaspoon maple syrup or sweetener of choice

½ tablespoon water

1 tablespoon pecans, roasted and crushed, or 1 tablespoon pecan butter, to serve

1   For the porridge, bring the water, salt and oats to the boil in a saucepan, turn down the heat to medium, add the milk and cook for about 4–5 minutes. Stir from time to time, ensuring that it doesn't stick to the bottom of the pan.

2   Mash the banana and add to the oats together with the maple syrup and vanilla extract. Stir well and cook for a further 4–5 minutes. Add another splash of milk if desired.

3   For the different fruit variations, heat the fruit together with the maple syrup and water in a saucepan and cook for a few minutes until softened.

4   Spoon the cooked fruit into a jar or bowl, followed by the cooked oats, and top with fresh fruit and nuts or nut butter.

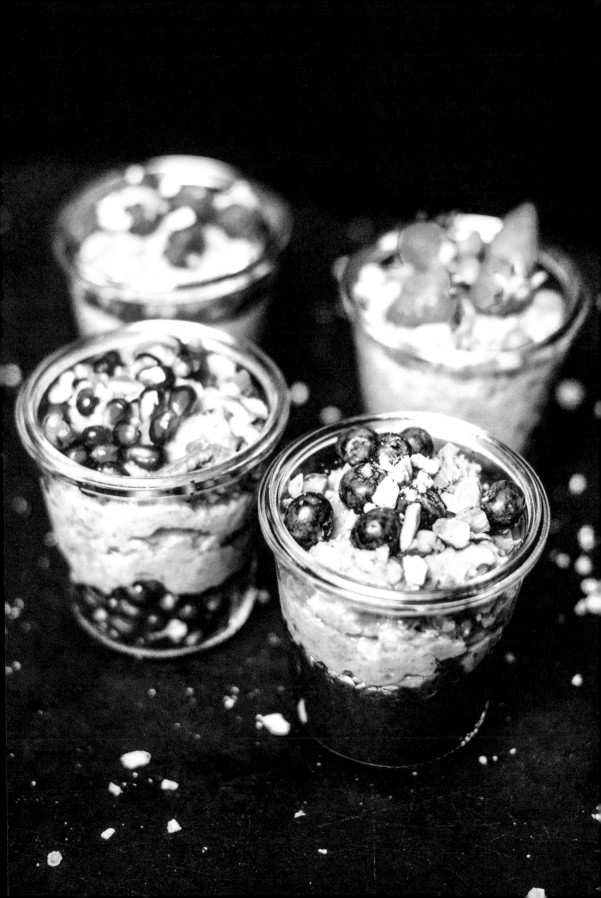

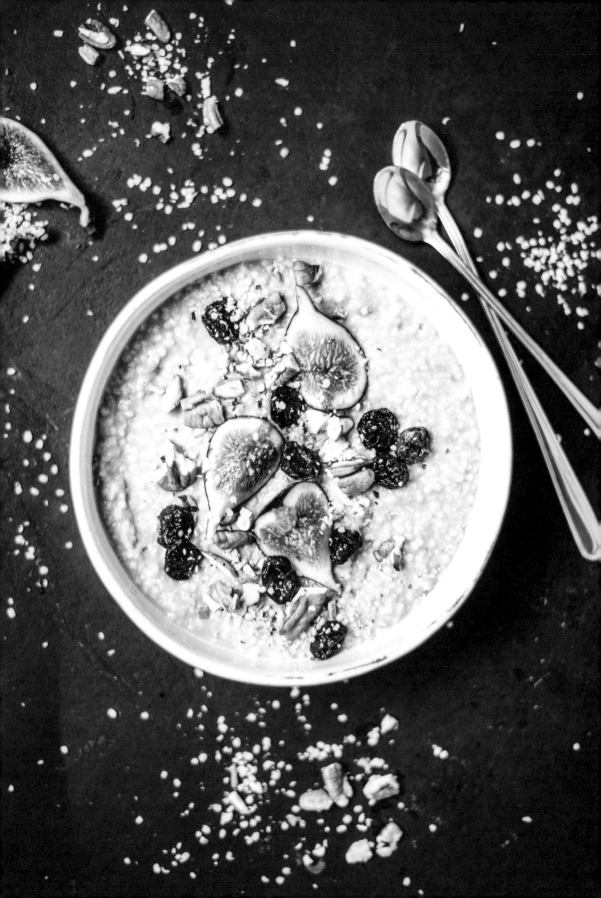

Cinnamon Millet Porridge with Fresh Figs, Cranberries & Roasted Nuts

A delicious hit of cinnamon.

Whether you enjoy this heart-warming breakfast on a cold winter morning or in the middle of summer, it's perfect to start the day off right. Not only filling, this porridge (oatmeal) will keep you energised throughout the day and make your tummy happy and satisfied. You've never had millet for breakfast before? Then it's about time you try it! Millet is one of my favourite wholegrains to make porridge with. And its delicious, nutty taste goes so well with cinnamon and figs.

SERVES 1 / GF, DF, VGN, RSF

PORRIDGE (OATMEAL)

200 ml (7 fl oz) water

pinch of salt

4 tablespoons millet

100 ml (3½ fl oz) milk of choice, e.g. soy, almond, rice milk

1 teaspoon ground cinnamon

2–3 teaspoon maple syrup or sweetener of choice

1 tablespoon almond butter

TOPPINGS

2 fresh figs

1 tablespoon dried unsweetened cranberries

2–3 teaspoons crushed pistachios, roasted

2–3 teaspoons crushed pecans, roasted

maple syrup or sweetener of choice

1   Bring the water and the salt to a boil, add the millet and cook in a saucepan over a medium heat for about 12–14 minutes.

2   Add the remaining ingredients, stir well, turn down the heat a bit and cook for another 4–5 minutes.

3   For the topping, put the crushed pistachios and pecans into a frying pan (skillet), drizzle some maple syrup on top and toast over a medium heat for a couple of minutes or until golden brown. Take off the heat and let them cool.

4   Add another dash of milk to the porridge if desired and pour into your breakfast bowl.

5   Cut the figs into quarters and arrange them on top of the porridge. Sprinkle over the cranberries and roasted nuts. If you like you can drizzle more maple syrup on top.

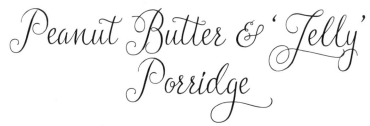

Peanut Butter & 'Jelly' Porridge

A mouthwatering combination from the USA.

I'm sure most of you have at least heard of the combination of peanut butter and jelly. In America, jelly is the same as jam in the UK and to know how good it actually tastes with peanut butter, you have to try it! A few years ago I lived in Canada for six months and was introduced to porridge creations that I had never encountered before. It took me four months to give the peanut butter and jelly combination a try and I have to admit, it's a real taste sensation! They belong together like Switzerland and chocolate and that says a lot. So please, try it as fast as you can and don't wait for four months.

SERVES 1 / (GF), DF, VGN, RSF

PORRIDGE (OATMEAL)
150 ml (5 fl oz) water

pinch of salt

4 tablespoons oats (gluten-free)

250 ml (8½ fl oz) milk of choice, e.g. soy, almond, rice milk

1 small ripe banana

2–3 teaspoons maple syrup or sweetener of choice

1 tablespoon peanut butter

'JELLY'
150 g (5 oz) berries of choice

1 teaspoon chia seeds

2–3 teaspoons maple syrup or sweetener of choice

1 tablespoon water

few drops of vanilla extract

TOPPINGS
strawberries

1–2 teaspoons peanut butter

crushed peanuts

1   For the 'jelly', bring all the ingredients to the boil in a saucepan, turn down the heat a bit and cook until the berries are softened. Take off the heat, stir well with a fork and set aside.

2   To make the porridge, bring the water, salt and oats to the boil in a saucepan, then reduce the heat.

3   Mash the banana with a fork and stir into the oats along with the milk, maple syrup and vanilla extract. Cook for about 5–7 minutes. Stir in the peanut butter, 1 tablespoon of the 'jelly' and another splash of milk if desired.

4   Pour the porridge into a bowl and top with fresh strawberries, peanut butter and some more 'jelly'. Sprinkle crushed peanuts on top.

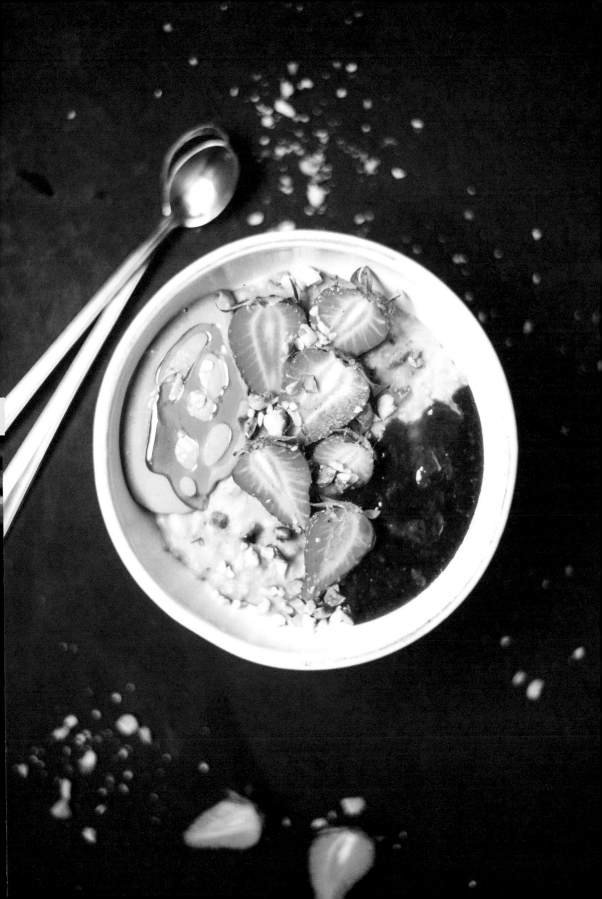

Mango, Banana & Peanut Trio on a Bed of Couscous

A sweet couscous breakfast — so fluffy and light.

The combination of mango, banana and peanut butter is incredibly tasty. When I first made this recipe I used cooked quinoa. I wanted to make it again but had run out of quinoa and thought of other wholegrains I could replace it with. Couscous is something I had only ever had in savoury dishes. It got me really excited to find out what it tasted like alongside sweet ingredients. This breakfast can be prepared the night before to save you time in the morning. Simply put it in the fridge overnight and grab it the next day. The flavours are enhanced when the dish is eaten cooled. For enough sweetness, it's important to use a very ripe mango and banana.

SERVES 1 / DF, VGN, RSF

COUSCOUS

100 ml (3½ fl oz) water

pinch of salt

3 tablespoons wheat couscous

1 teaspoon coconut oil

100–150 ml (3½–5 fl oz) milk of choice, e.g. soy, almond, rice milk

few drops of vanilla extract

2 teaspoons maple syrup or sweetener of choice

TOPPING

1 ripe banana

dash of milk of choice, e.g. soy, almond, rice milk

2–3 teaspoons peanut butter

1 teaspoons maple syrup or sweetener of choice

1 ripe mango

roasted and crushed peanuts

1   Bring the water and salt to the boil in a lidded saucepan. Add the couscous and coconut oil, stir well, cook for 2 minutes, then take off the heat. Cover with the lid and leave it to swell for a few minutes.

2   Meanwhile, prepare the toppings. In a bowl, mash the banana with a fork, add a dash of milk, the peanut butter and maple syrup and stir until well combined.

3   Peel the mango and cut into small cubes. Add half of it to the banana mixture and give it a good stir until the mango has softened and is slightly mashed.

4   Add the milk, vanilla extract and maple syrup to the couscous and loosen up the grains with a fork. Transfer the couscous into a bowl or deep plate.

5   Top the couscous with the banana and mango mash and garnish with the remaining mango cubes. Sprinkle the crushed peanuts on top and add another splash of milk for a bit more moisture, if desired.

VARIATIONS   If you don't like couscous you can replace it with quinoa, amaranth or millet. However, they all have a longer cooking time.

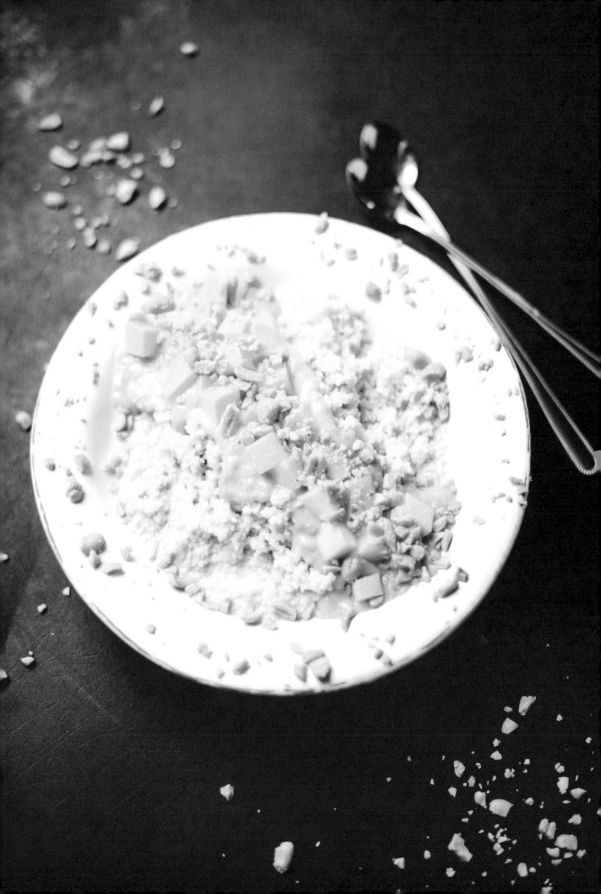

Power Food Chia Porridge with Hot Berries

Everything to satisfy you, packed into one breakfast.

It's absolutely worth getting up 10 minutes earlier in the morning to make this delicious porridge (oatmeal). Oats are one of the best things you can have for breakfast. They will keep you full, taste great eaten in a variety of ways and are a real power food. Chia seeds provide plenty of energy and good nutrients. The hot berries on top are rich in vitamins and antioxidants. To enhance the nutty taste and improve the texture, I love adding a splash of almond or rice milk over the cooked oats.

SERVES 1 / (GF), DF, VGN, RSF

PORRIDGE (OATMEAL)

250 ml (8½ fl oz) water

pinch of salt

70 g (2½ oz/generous ½ cup) oats (oatmeal) (gluten-free)

1 tablespoon chia seeds

200 ml (7 fl oz) milk of choice, e.g. soy, almond, rice milk

2–3 teaspoons maple syrup or sweetener of choice

few drops of pure vanilla extract

TOPPINGS

200 g (7 oz) fresh or frozen mixed berries

1 teaspoon maple syrup or sweetener of choice

2–3 teaspoons almond butter

a splash of milk of choice, e.g. soy, almond, rice milk etc.

crushed nuts of choice

handful of fresh blueberries

1   Bring the water and salt to the boil in a saucepan, add the oats and chia seeds and cook over a medium heat for about 2–3 minutes. Slowly pour in the milk, add the maple syrup and vanilla extract and cook for another 4–5 minutes. Stir from time to time.

2   For the topping, heat up the berries together with the sweetener in a small saucepan on medium heat. Cook for a few minutes until softened.

3   Spoon the cooked chia porridge into a bowl and add the hot berries on top, along with all the berry juice from the pan.

4   With a fork, mix the almond butter well with the milk and maple syrup until smooth and drizzle on top of the porridge. Sprinkle over the crushed nuts. I personally love adding some fresh blueberries on top as well because they provide some extra sweetness and, of course, energy.

TIP   This recipe can be prepared the night before, ready for you to grab as a breakfast to-go. Or you can even prepare it in the morning, bring it with you for lunch and start the afternoon full of energy. Simply store it in a sealed jar in the fridge and sprinkle the nuts on top right before eating so that they keep their crunchiness.

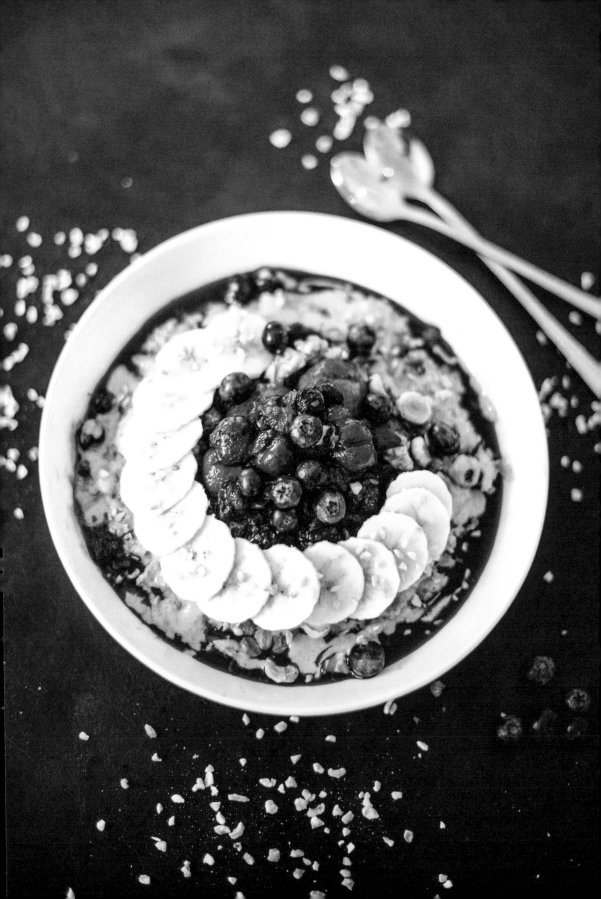

Millet & Oat Porridge with Caramelised Banana

A porridge you need to try!

Mmmm, I can still remember the smell when I first made this recipe – it filled the whole apartment and pulled my sister right out of bed. I do use a lot of bananas in my recipes, especially for breakfast, but this caramelised banana takes it to another level. The banana is caramelised with coconut sugar and I did the same with some shredded coconut and pecans. The flavour that came out was simply magical. A breakfast that never gets boring and would never fail to amaze me, even if I had to eat it three times a day!

SERVES 1-2 / (GF), DF, VGN, RSF

PORRIDGE (OATMEAL)

250 ml (8½ fl oz) water

pinch of salt

2–3 tablespoons millet flakes

2–3 tablespoons oats (oatmeal) (gluten-free)

250 ml (8½ fl oz) milk of choice, e.g. soy, almond, rice milk

1 tablespoon coconut oil

2–3 teaspoons coconut nectar or coconut sugar

TOPPINGS

1 banana

1 teaspoon coconut oil

1 tablespoon shredded coconut

6–8 pecans

2–3 teaspoons coconut sugar

coconut nectar, to serve

1   Make the porridge by bringing the water and salt to the boil in a saucepan. Add the oats and millet flakes and cook over a medium heat for 2–3 minutes. Slowly add the milk, then add the coconut oil and coconut nectar or sugar. Stir well and cook for about 5 minutes, stirring occasionally.

2   For the caramelised banana, heat up the coconut oil in a small frying pan (skillet) over a medium heat. Halve the banana lengthwise and place in the pan with the cut side down. Reduce the heat a bit.

3   Sprinkle the shredded coconut over the banana slices, add the pecans into the pan and sprinkle the coconut sugar on top. After 2–3 minutes, turn the banana slices over and caramelise on the other side for 2–3 more minutes. Take off the heat.

4   Pour the porridge into a bowl and place the caramelised banana slices and pecans on top. Drizzle some coconut nectar over everything, enjoy the beautiful aroma and dig in!

VARIATIONS   If you don't have millet flakes to hand you can either replace them with quinoa flakes or just use oats.

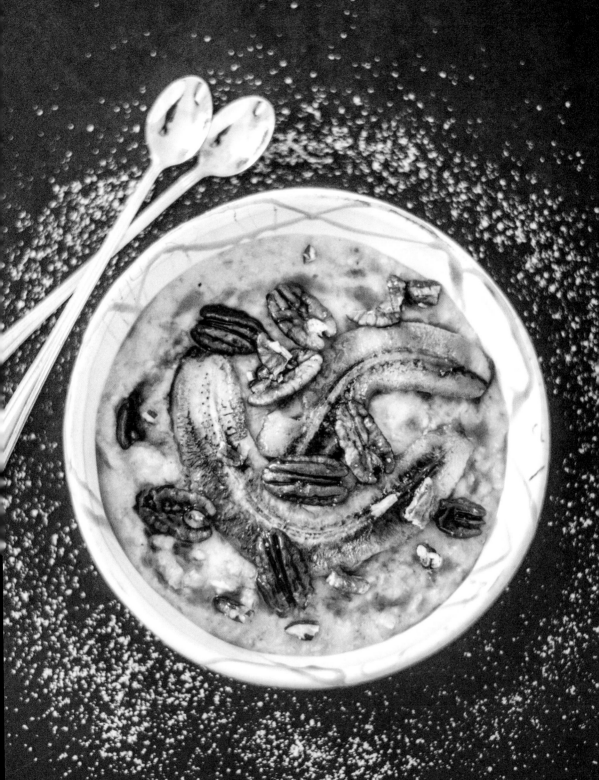

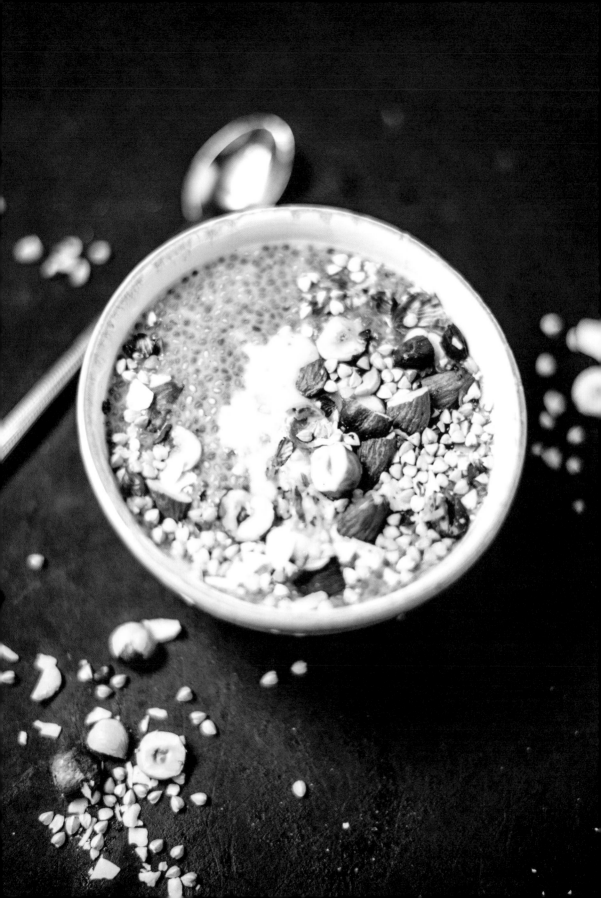

Almond Milk Chia Pudding with Roasted Nuts

This chia pudding drives me nuts – but in a really good way!

This chia pudding is perfect as a snack or light breakfast. It contains healthy fats from the nuts, and chia seeds contain a lot of iron. Using roasted nuts will bring out the flavour a lot more, so don't leave this step out. Roasted nuts are not only better in taste, but also easier to crush. Because the whole process of roasting nuts takes about 20 minutes until they're cooled and ready to eat, I usually buy large quantities of different kinds of nuts and roast them all at once. I then store them in sealed jars so that I have roasted nuts on hand whenever I need them.

SERVES 1 / GF, DF, VGN, RSF

CHIA PUDDING

3 tablespoons chia seeds

300 ml (10 fl oz) almond milk or milk of choice

1 vanilla bean, seeds scraped

2–3 teaspoons maple syrup or sweetener of choice

1 ripe banana

2–3 teaspoons almond or peanut butter

TOPPINGS

1 tablespoon puffed quinoa

1–2 tablespoons roasted and crushed nuts of choice

nut butter of choice (optional)

1   Add the chia seeds, milk, vanilla seeds and maple syrup into a lidded jar and stir well. Mash the banana with a fork, add to the chia seeds together with the nut butter and stir again until well combined. Soak overnight or for at least 2 hours in the fridge.

2   Take the chia pudding out of the fridge and stir well to break up any lumps. Pour into a bowl, top with the puffed quinoa and roasted nuts and drizzle over some nut butter if desired.

Coconut Chia Pudding with Blackberry Sauce & Passion Fruit

An alternative consistency combined with great taste – a real food experience!
I had chia pudding for the first time not too long ago. Even though the consistency
was completely new to me, I loved it from the beginning. It's amazing how much
the chia seeds expand after soaking them. Before soaking, it's important that you mix
them really well with the milk. And before serving the pudding into your bowl make
sure you stir again to avoid lumps. You can add the blackberry sauce on top either still
warm or cold, whatever you prefer. Don't forget the passion fruit –
it gives the dish an extra special, fruity taste.

SERVES 1 / GF, DF, VGN, RSF

CHIA PUDDING

3 tablespoons chia seeds

250–300 ml (8½–10 fl oz) coconut milk

2 teaspoons maple syrup or sweetener
  of choice

1 ripe banana

BLACKBERRY SAUCE

200 g (8 oz/1½ cups) fresh or frozen
  blackberries

2 tablespoons water

2 teaspoons maple syrup or sweetener
  of choice

few drops of vanilla extract

TOPPINGS

fresh blackberries

fresh blueberries

unsweetened coconut chips

2 ripe passion fruit

1   First make the chia pudding. In a large bowl, mix together
the chia seeds, milk and maple syrup. Mash the banana with
a fork in a separate bowl, add to the chia seeds and stir well.
Leave to soak overnight in the fridge or for a minimum of
2 hours.

2   For the blackberry sauce, add the blackberries, water,
maple syrup and vanilla extract into a small saucepan. Cook
over a medium heat until softened.

3   Take the chia pudding out of the fridge and stir well to
break up any lumps. Pour into a bowl and top with the
blackberry sauce, fresh berries, coconut chips and
passion fruit.

TIP   If you don't like bananas or aren't really hungry, you
can leave them out. I personally prefer having chia pudding
with banana because it not only adds some extra natural
sweetness, but also provides plenty of energy and keeps you
full for longer. The choice is totally up to you.

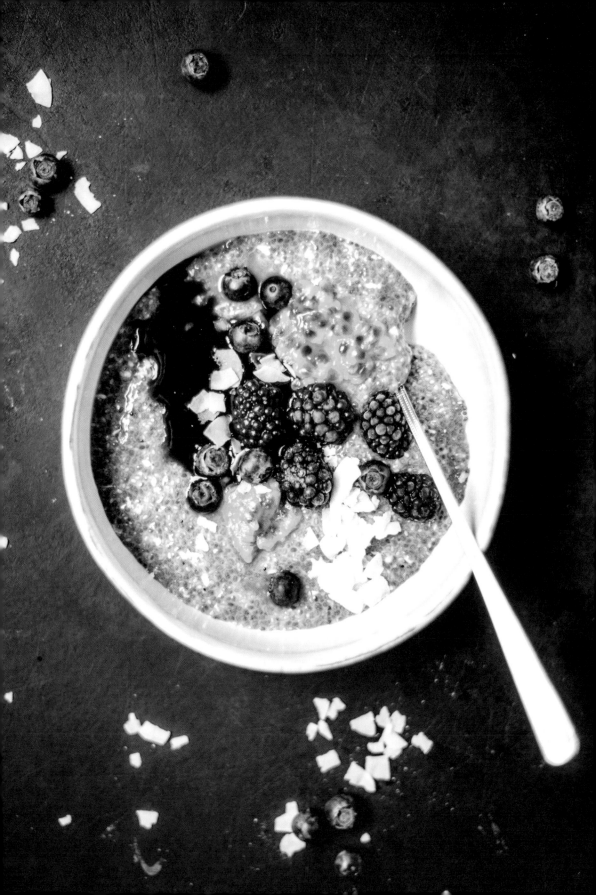

Creamy Amaranth Porridge with Raspberry Coulis

A breakfast to float you up to Cloud Nine.

What an extremely creamy and heart-warming breakfast that brings the whole family to the table and makes everybody want to have the last spoonful. Even though it's light and fruity, it keeps you full for some time. The warm raspberries go so well together with the amaranth porridge and passion fruit, and they balance out the flavours of the different ingredients with their slight tartness. Since amaranth has a pretty long cooking time, you can either prepare it the night before or get up early and do a little home workout while it's cooking. Then you absolutely deserve every single spoonful of it!

SERVES 2 / GF, DF, VGN, RSF

PORRIDGE (OATMEAL)

250–300 ml (8½–10 fl oz) water

pinch of salt

8 tablespoons amaranth

200–250 ml (7–8½ fl oz) milk of choice, e.g. soy, almond, rice milk

2–3 teaspoons maple syrup or sweetener of choice

1 vanilla bean, seeds scraped

RASPBERRY COULIS

300 g (10½ oz/2½ cups) fresh or frozen raspberries

1–2 teaspoons maple syrup or sweetener of choice

TOPPINGS

2 passion fruit

2 handfuls of fresh raspberries

12–16 roasted and crushed pistachios

1   To make the amaranth porridge, bring the water and salt to the boil in a saucepan, add the amaranth and cook over a high heat for about 1 minute. Turn down the heat and let it cook over a low heat for 18–20 minutes, stirring from time to time. Gradually stir in the milk. Add the maple syrup and vanilla seeds, stir well, and take the pan off the heat, Cover with a lid and leave to swell for about 15 minutes.

2   For the raspberry coulis, put both the raspberries and maple syrup into a saucepan, add a splash of water and cook for about 5 minutes until the berries are soft. Pour the raspberry coulis into deep dishes or bowls.

3   Add a splash more milk to the amaranth porridge and, if desired, heat it up again very quickly. Stir well, then pour on top of the raspberry coulis. Garnish with passion fruit and fresh raspberries, then sprinkle the crushed pistachios on top.

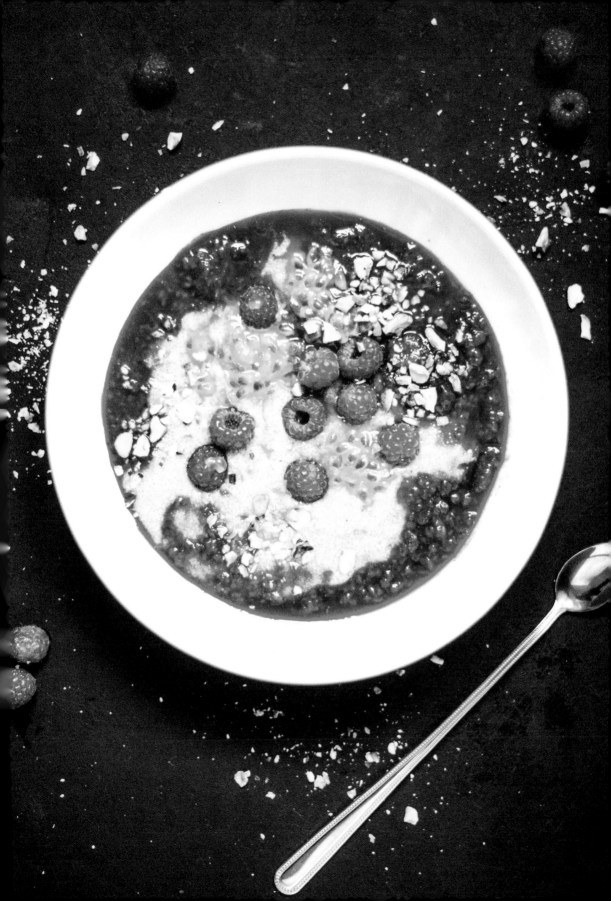

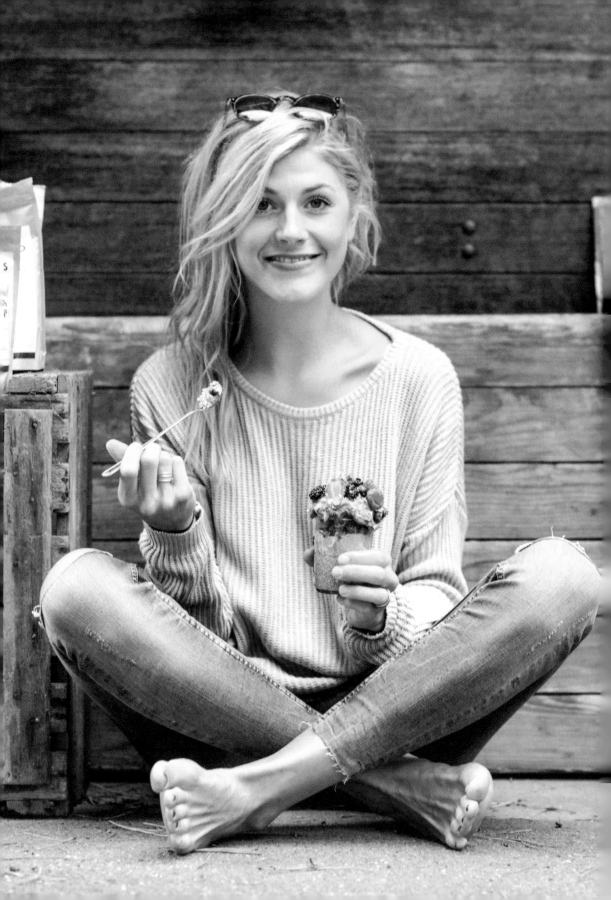

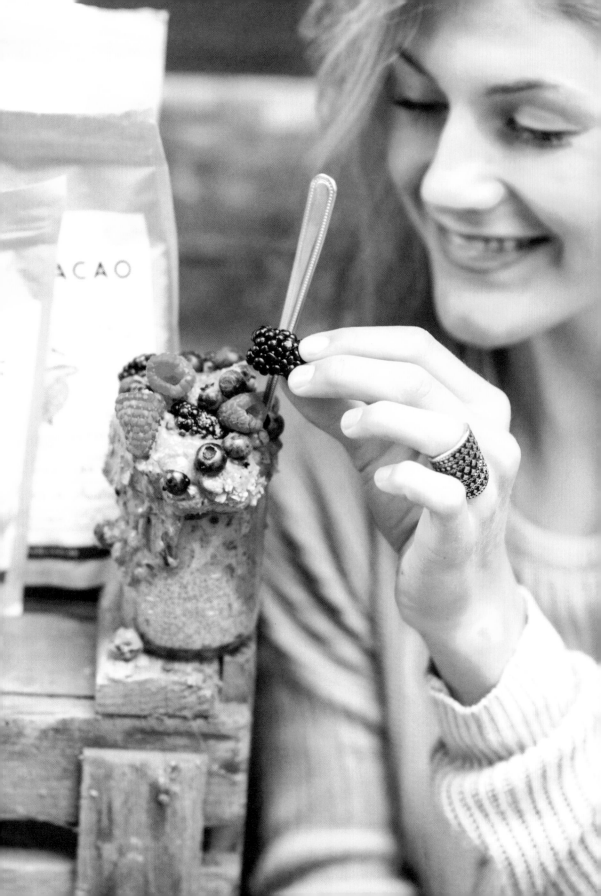

Peanut Butter & Oat Shake

Something I can't get enough of!
Whenever I don't have a lot of time in the morning, I usually make this shake.
It's not only super filling, but also incredibly tasty. I'm a real peanut fan and therefore love
to make my own peanut butter with no added sugar or fats. Feel free to use your
preferred milk for this recipe. I tried it with quite a few different kinds of milk and,
personally, I think that oat milk, spelt drink or rice milk go really well with it.
If you prepare this shake to take away, pour it into a lidded jar, store it in the fridge
and shake well before drinking. Kids love this shake as well!

SERVES 1 (OR 2 AS A SNACK) / (GF), DF, VGN, RSF

1 tablespoon peanut butter

300 ml (10 fl oz) milk of choice, e.g. oat, almond, rice milk

2–3 teaspoons maple syrup or sweetener of choice

3 tablespoons oats (oatmeal) (gluten-free)

1 banana, sliced

1   Add all the ingredients into a blender and blend for about 4–5 minutes until smooth and creamy.

2   Pour the shake into a jar and enjoy right away or store in the fridge with the lid on until you're ready to drink it.

TIP   You can enjoy this shake in two servings as a snack after a workout or simply if you need some energy.

VARIATIONS   Use frozen banana slices for a more refreshing shake. For those who don't like bananas or want something slightly lighter, simply leave the banana out and add a couple of Medjool dates instead.

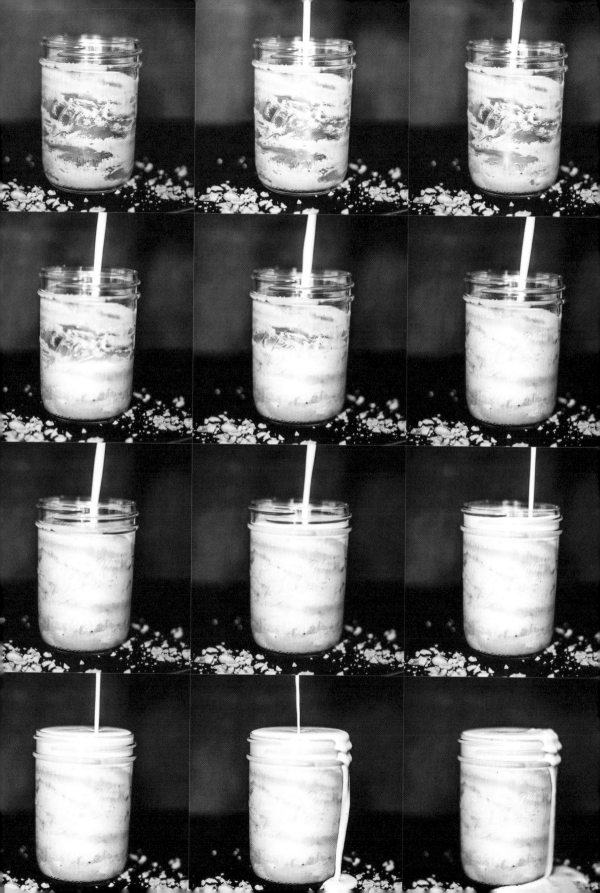

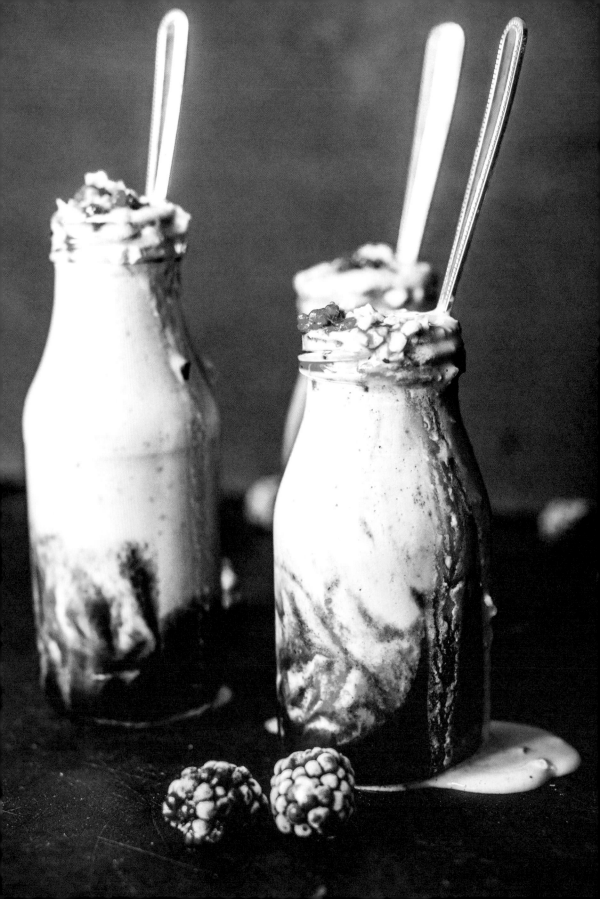

Blackberry & Raspberry Shake

You can never have too many berries!
Every time I bite into a fresh, juicy and sweet berry, I am reminded of how much
I love them. For this recipe you can use fresh or frozen berries.
Berries are rich in antioxidants and very low in calories compared to other fruits.
This shake puts you in a good mood in no time and is an eye-catcher at any brunch,
party or served as a refreshing dessert for friends and family.

——— SERVES 1 (OR 2-3 AS A SNACK) / GF, DF*, VGN*, RSF ———

SHAKE

150 g (5 oz) fresh or frozen
  blackberries

150 g (5 oz) fresh or frozen
  raspberries

2 teaspoons maple syrup or sweetener
  of choice

3–4 tablespoons water

150 ml (5 fl oz) milk of choice, e.g. soy,
  almond, rice milk

1 vanilla bean, seeds scraped

200 g (7 oz) Greek yoghurt or *soy yoghurt

2 teaspoons maple syrup or sweetener of
  choice

splash of fresh lemon juice

TOPPINGS

crushed nuts of choice

fresh berries

1   Blend 50 g (2 oz) of both the blackberries and raspberries with the water and maple syrup to a smooth and creamy consistency. Pour into a jar or 2–3 small glasses.

2   Add all the remaining ingredients into a blender and blend until smooth.

3   Pour the yoghurt mixture on top of the berry purée and sprinkle some crushed nuts and berries on top. Best enjoyed right away!

TIP   If you want the shake to be a little more liquid, add another splash of milk. To make the swirl pattern, use a long spoon, go all the way to the bottom of the jar and make a few circles halfway up and along the glasses.

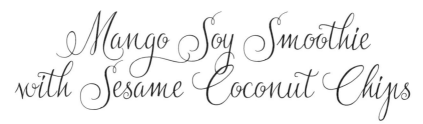

Mango Soy Smoothie with Sesame Coconut Chips

The best and easiest mango smoothie.
This smoothie, topped with the crispy coconut chips, satisfies my taste buds every time.
It's important to use very sweet and almost overripe mangoes. I suggest that you use soy
yoghurt rather than any other type because it harmonises really well with the mango and
honey. The coconut chips can be made in no time and provide the required crunch.
A recipe that will win over breakfast newcomers, dessert lovers
and even those who think they are already full.

SERVES 2-3 / GF, DF, VGN, RSF

SESAME COCONUT CHIPS

2 tablespoons white sesame seeds

2–3 teaspoons rice syrup or sweetener
of choice

few drops of vanilla extract

100 g (3½ oz) unsweetened coconut chips

SMOOTHIE

2 very ripe mangoes

400 g (14 oz) unsweetened soy yoghurt

1–1½ tablespoons maple syrup or sweetener
of choice

TOPPINGS

redcurrants or berries of choice

1   Preheat the oven to 160°C (320°F/Gas 3) and line a
baking sheet with parchment paper.

2   Start by making the sesame coconut chips. In a bowl,
mix the sesame seeds with the rice syrup and vanilla, then
add the coconut chips and mix with your hands until the
coconut chips are completely coated. Spread onto the baking
sheet and bake for about 15 minutes until golden brown.
Keep an eye on them, as they burn very easily. Once golden,
take the chips out of the oven and let them cool completely
so that they get crispy.

3   For the smoothie, peel the mangoes and cut them into
small pieces. Put them into the blender with the soy yoghurt
and maple syrup and blend for 3–4 minutes to a smooth,
creamy and slightly thick consistency. If you prefer a
thinner consistency, add a splash of soy milk.

4   Pour the mango soy smoothie into bowls, top with a
handful or two of the crispy coconut chips and garnish with
the berries.

TIPS   Use frozen mango pieces or blend some ice with the
mango and soy yoghurt if you want the smoothie to be even
more refreshing. The sesame coconut chips are very
addictive and will be finished pretty fast. If you have some
left, store the remaining coconut chips in an airtight jar and
keep for 4–5 days. Use as a topping for smoothies, shakes
and creams, or have a handful as a little snack.

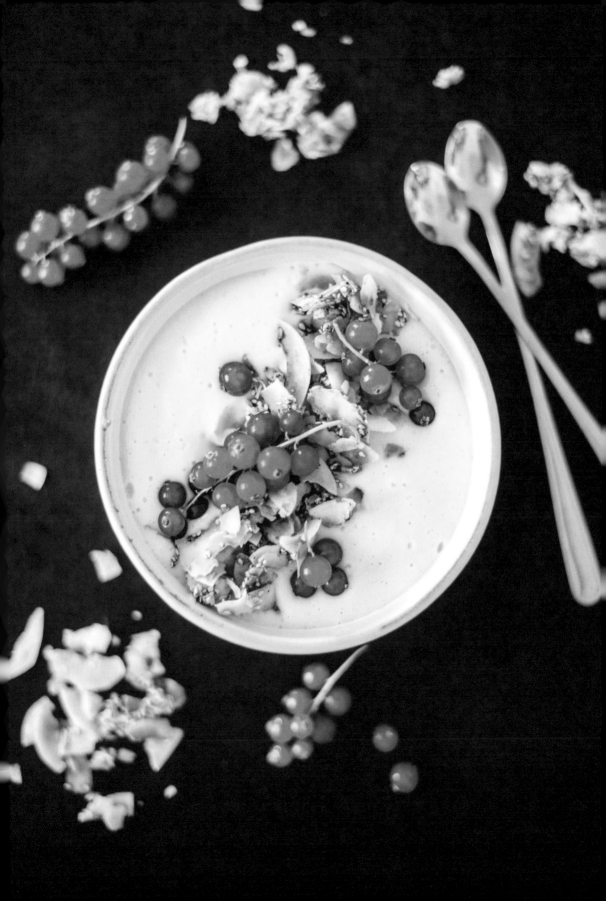

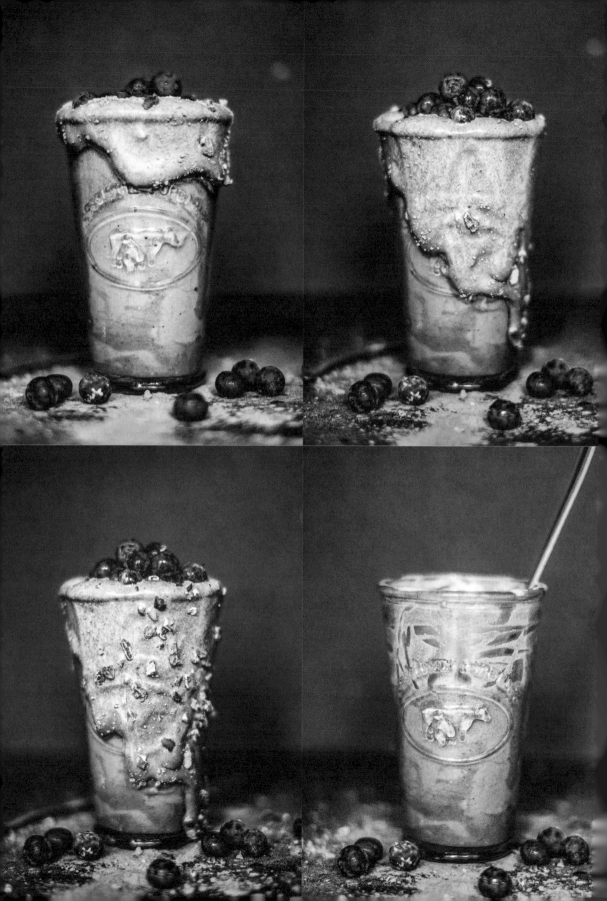

Sinfully Sweet Cacao Shake

Perfect to fuel up after a workout.

I love this shake after an intense workout! It's a real explosion of taste and texture. The protein powder helps your muscles to regenerate, and the banana and oats contain good carbohydrates that will help fill up your glycogen stores. This completely guilt-free shake tastes just like chocolate! You wouldn't believe that there is no chocolate or sugar in it at all. I hope that you now know what to treat yourself with after your next workout. If you tell yourself you can only drink this shake after doing a workout, you'll be working out every day – that's how delicious it is!

SERVES 1-2 / (GF), RSF

SHAKE

250 ml (8½ fl oz) milk of choice, e.g. soy, almond, rice milk

2 tablespoons raw cacao powder

1–2 tablespoons sugar-free protein powder (whey protein isolate), e.g. chocolate, natural, vanilla

1 banana, sliced and frozen

2 tablespoons oats (oatmeal) (gluten-free)

2 teaspoons peanut butter

few drops of vanilla extract

2–3 teaspoons maple syrup or sweetener of choice

100 ml (3½ fl oz) water

2 dates, pitted and soaked

TOPPINGS

2–3 teaspoons cacao nibs

berries of choice

1   Put all the ingredients for the shake into a blender and blend until you have a smooth and creamy consistency.

2   Pour the thick shake into a glass, sprinkle the cacao nibs on top, garnish with fresh berries and enjoy with a spoon or simply drink it. Alternatively, refrigerate until ready to drink.

PROTEIN POWDER   I always use organic sugar-free protein powder. If you don't have any protein powder at home, or don't necessarily want to buy some, replace it with another spoon of raw cacao powder. Raw cacao powder can be quite bitter though, so you might have to sweeten the shake a little bit more. Simply experiment and see what works best for you.

CACAO NIBS   These peeled and crushed cocoa beans are available in most health food stores or can be ordered online. They have a slightly bitter taste, just like very dark chocolate.

VARIATIONS   If you're vegan or want to make this shake dairy-free, simply use another protein powder such as soy protein powder and, of course, a plant-based milk.

Blueberry, Mint & Yoghurt Smoothie

Blue meets green and they fall in love.

Whenever it's hot outside, all I long for is a cold, refreshing and fruity smoothie. I love to try out new flavour combinations. I did just that in this recipe by marrying blueberries and mint. The yoghurt makes the smoothie incredibly creamy. Feel free to use fresh or frozen berries. If you use frozen berries simply thaw them for a few minutes first. A must-try smoothie to enjoy in summer or to kick-start the day in the right way.

—————————— SERVES 1 GF, DF*, VGN*, RSF ——————————

FOR THE SMOOTHIE

250 g (9 oz) fresh or frozen blueberries

10–12 mint leaves

2–3 teaspoons maple syrup or sweetener of choice

100–150 ml (3½–5 fl oz) milk of choice, e.g. soy, almond, rice milk

250 g (9 oz) low-fat yoghurt or *soy yoghurt

few drops of vanilla extract

2 teaspoons almond butter

TOPPINGS

mint leaves

fresh blueberries

1   Put all of the ingredients into a blender and blend until creamy. Add more mint leaves if you would like an extra minty flavour.

2   Pour the shake into a jar, garnish with some fresh mint leaves and serve with fresh blueberries. Either enjoy right away or cool in the fridge for about 30 minutes.

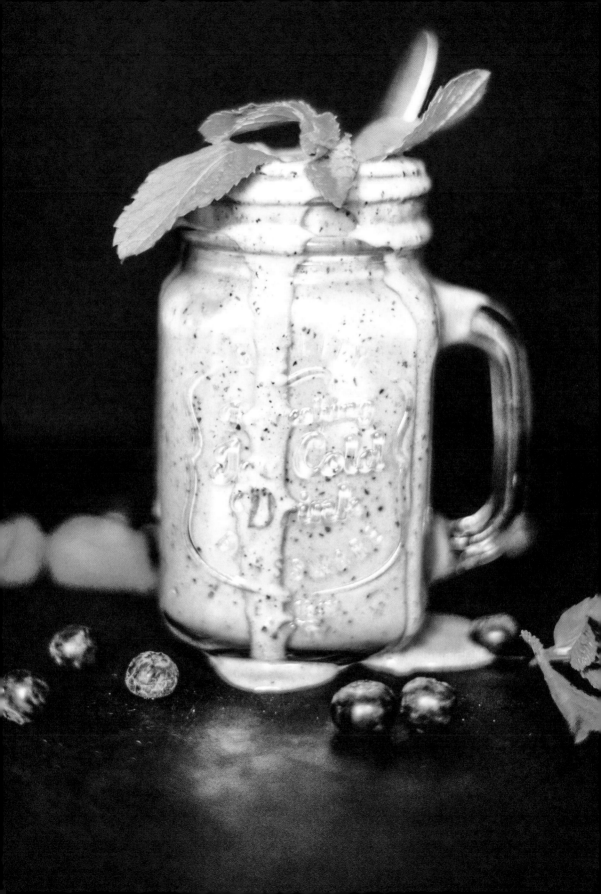

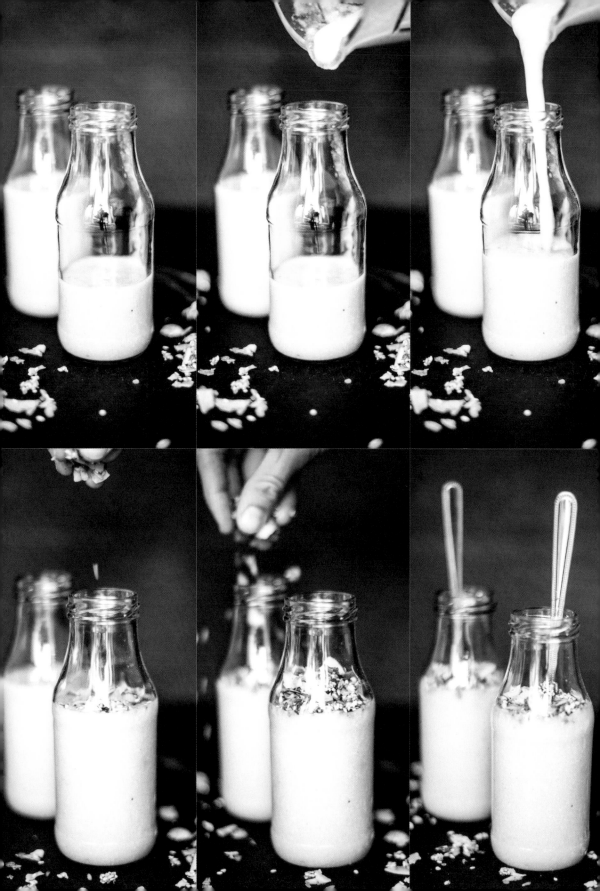

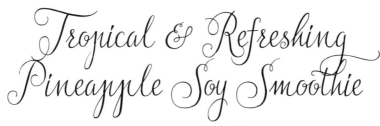

Tropical & Refreshing Pineapple Soy Smoothie

An exotic start to the day.

You can't beat a fresh, ripe, sweet and juicy pineapple. This smoothie guarantees
a good mood and is reminiscent of holidays, sun and fun. It's really important to use
a ripe pineapple for this recipe. Even though the smoothie has enough sweetness already
from the pineapple and banana, a teaspoon of honey can never hurt
and will intensify the sweet flavour even more.

SERVES 1 (OR 2-3 AS A SNACK) / GF, DF, VGN, RSF

SMOOTHIE

1 small ripe pineapple (about 400 g/14 oz)

1 banana, sliced and frozen

150–200 ml (5–7 fl oz) milk of choice,
e.g. soy, almond, rice milk

120 g (4 oz) soy yoghurt

2 tablespoons shredded coconut or
1 tablespoon coconut butter

1 teaspoon maple syrup or sweetener
of choice

TOPPING

2 tablespoons Sesame Coconut Chips
(see page 96)

1   Peel the pineapple, halve the fruit lengthwise, remove
the core and cut into pieces.

2   Put the pineapple chunks and all the remaining
ingredients into a blender and blend to a smooth and creamy
consistency.

3   Pour the smoothie into a jar or a few smaller glasses,
add some sesame coconut chips on top and enjoy.

Crunchy Cinnamon Granola with Banana & Cinnamon Milk

The proof that granola is so much better when home-made!
I love it when the smell of freshly baked granola fills the whole apartment. When it is
fresh out of the oven, it not only tastes the best, but that's also when it is crunchiest.
There are so many different kinds of granola to choose from at the supermarket – too
many in my opinion, which makes it difficult to decide which variety to get.
Refined sugar and other preservatives are hidden in most of them. That's why you should
make the granola yourself. It's super easy, quick to make and you know exactly what's in
it. The banana and cinnamon milk welcomes you to a completely new granola experience
and adds a delicious sweet taste. A great recipe to serve for
a weekend brunch with your loved ones.

SERVES 4-5 / (GF), DF, VGN, RSF

CINNAMON GRANOLA

150 g (5 oz/1½ cups) oats (oatmeal)
   (gluten-free)

6 tablespoons pumpkin seeds

4 tablespoons sunflower seeds

4 tablespoons almonds, crushed

1 teaspoon cinnamon

pinch of salt

2 tablespoons hemp hearts (see page 31)

1 ripe banana

1½ teaspoons rice syrup or maple syrup

1 tablespoon nut butter of choice

1½ tablespoons coconut oil, melted

few drops of vanilla extract

BANANA & CINNAMON MILK

2 ripe bananas

150 ml (5 fl oz) water

100 ml (3½ fl oz) milk of choice, e.g. soy,
   almond, rice milk

4–5 dates, pitted, or 3 Medjool dates

½ teaspoon cinnamon

few drops of vanilla extract

TOPPINGS

fresh berries of choice

1   Preheat the oven to 170°C (340°F/Gas 3½) and line a
baking tray with parchment paper.

2   For the granola, add the oats, seeds, almonds, cinnamon,
salt and hemp hearts into a bowl and mix with a spoon. In
a separate bowl, mash the banana, then add the remaining
wet ingredients and mix well. Pour the banana mixture into
the dry mixture. Stir well and spread it out evenly on the
baking sheet.

3   Bake the granola for about 20 minutes, then remove
from the oven and loosen up with a spoon so that it browns
evenly. Bake for another 20 minutes. Take it out of the oven
and let it cool completely.

4   For the banana and cinnamon milk, blend all the
ingredients to a light and creamy consistency for about
3 minutes and put it in the fridge while the granola cools.
Give it a good stir or blend again before serving.

5   Enjoy the granola with the banana and cinnamon milk
and fresh berries. I love using strawberries here, or fruit
such as fresh mango or baked apple pieces.

STORAGE   You can keep the granola in a sealed jar for up
to 1–2 weeks, although it's best and crunchiest eaten fresh.
The banana and cinnamon milk is also a delicious drink by
itself. It tastes great with 3 tablespoons of oats blended in
– perfect for breakfast or a post-workout drink.

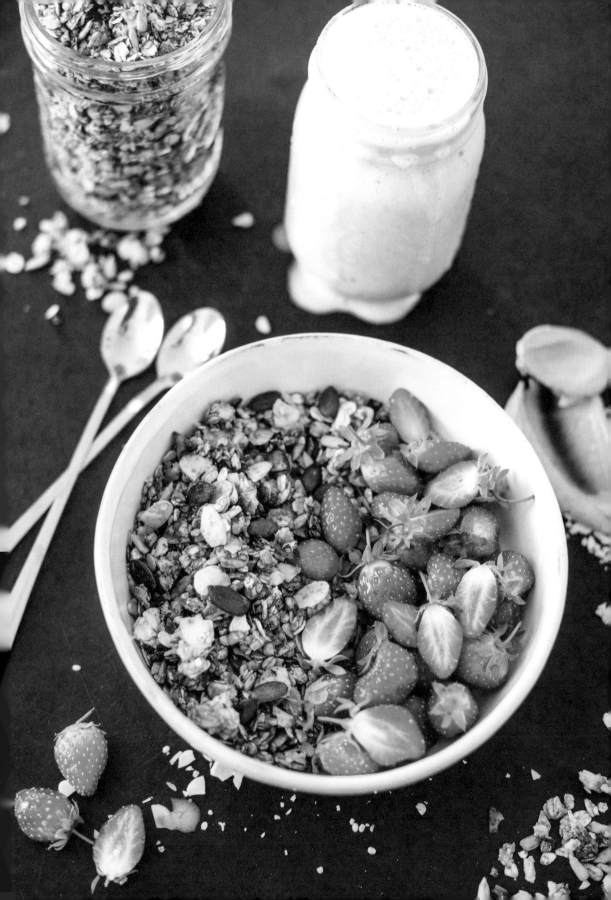

Spelt Waffles with Almond & Berry Cream

Get the waffle iron on as fast as you can!

Most of you probably love waffles and so do I. Back when I was a child, we used to eat so many of them with plenty of icing (confectioner's) sugar on top. With this recipe you can enjoy eating waffles without feeling guilty at all. And once you've tried this almond and berry cream, I promise you, you will quickly forget about icing sugar.

———————— SERVES 2 (APPROX. 4 WAFFLES) / RSF ————————

WAFFLES

4 tablespoons wholemeal spelt flour

1 teaspoon baking powder

pinch of salt

4 tablespoons oats (oatmeal) (gluten-free)

100 ml (3½ fl oz) milk of choice, e.g. soy, almond, rice milk

1 egg

1 ripe banana

2 teaspoons coconut oil, plus extra for greasing

2 teaspoons maple syrup or sweetener of choice

1 tablespoon almond butter

ALMOND & BERRY CREAM

4 tablespoons soy yoghurt

1 tablespoon almond butter

2–3 teaspoons maple syrup or sweetener of choice

few drops of vanilla extract

3–4 tablespoons mixed berries

2 tablespoons water

TOPPINGS

fresh berries

almonds, roasted and crushed

1   To make the waffles, put the spelt flour, baking powder and salt into a bowl and stir well. Blend the remaining ingredients in a food processor until smooth, then add to the flour mixture and carefully stir with a whisk or fork into a smooth dough. Let it rest for about 10 minutes.

2   For the almond and berry cream, mix the soy yoghurt, almond butter, 1–2 teaspoons of the maple syrup and the vanilla extract to a creamy consistency.

3   Heat up the berries with the water and 1 teaspoon of the maple syrup in a small saucepan and cook over a medium heat for a few minutes. Take off the heat and purée until smooth. Pour it on top of the almond cream and give it a quick swirl.

4   Heat up the waffle iron and grease with coconut oil. Add 2 tablespoons of the waffle mixture for each waffle and fry on both sides until golden brown.

5   Put the waffles onto a plate and enjoy with some of the almond cream and fresh berries on top. For the perfect crunch, sprinkle some roasted and crushed almonds on top.

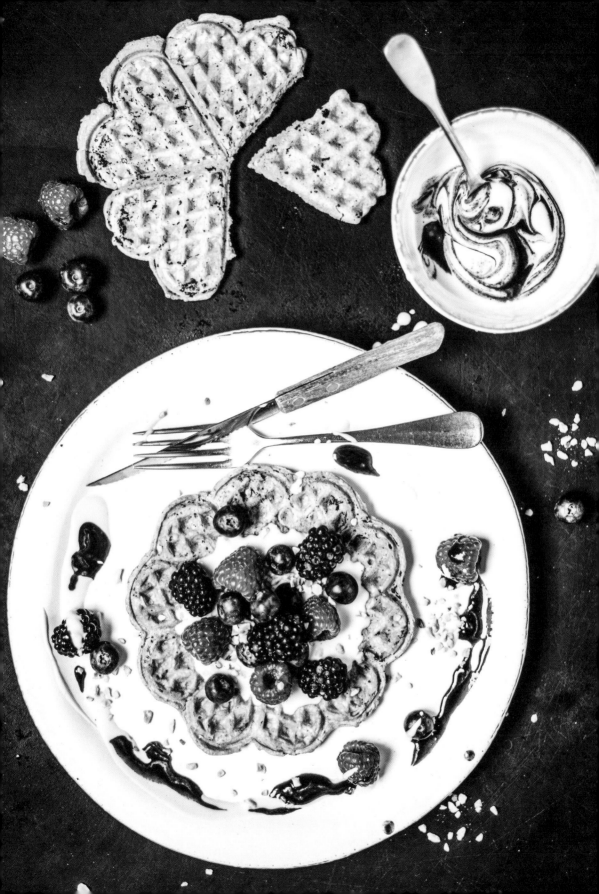

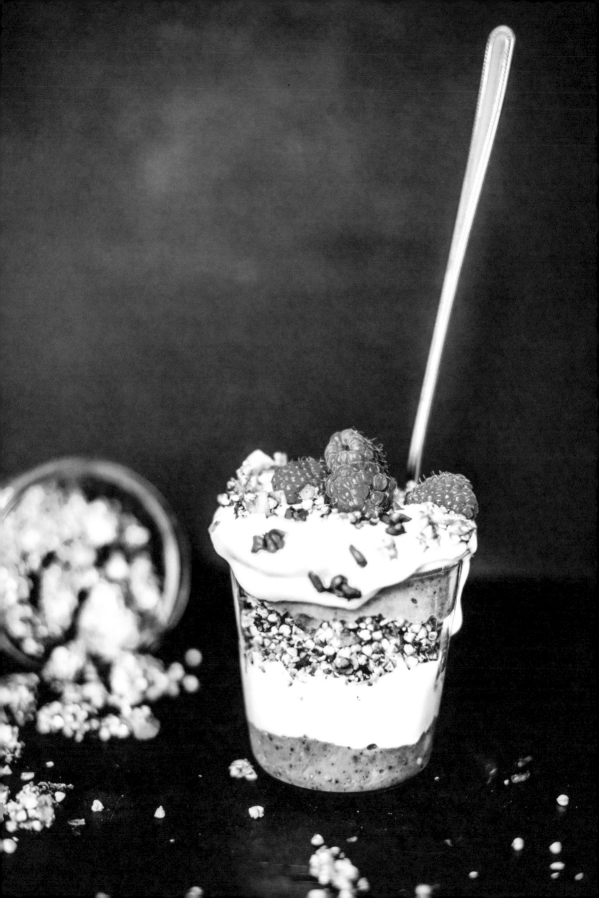

Rhubarb & Peach Compote with Buckwheat Granola

Bittersweet, creamy, crunchy, fruity – all in one jar.
This jarful of deliciousness assures a good start to the day and brings colour and life to afternoon tea with friends. Both the taste and the look will impress your guests. The granola is gluten-free, crunchy and very easy to make. This recipe will make a big batch of granola, which you can store and have with almond milk and fresh fruit, or sprinkle some on top of your smoothie.

SERVES 3-4 / GF, DF*, VGN*, RSF

GRANOLA

2 ripe bananas

1 tablespoon maple syrup or sweetener of choice

1 tablespoon coconut oil, melted

1 vanilla bean, seeds scraped

pinch of salt

250 g (9 oz) buckwheat

100 g (3½ oz) quinoa flakes or oats (oatmeal) (gluten-free)

100 g (3½ oz) unsweetened coconut chips

2 teaspoons maca powder

150 g (5 oz) sesame seeds

RHUBARB COMPOTE

400 g (14 oz) red rhubarb

2 ripe peaches

4 tablespoons water

1 teaspoon lemon juice

1 teaspoon vanilla extract

4–5 teaspoons maple syrup or sweetener of choice

200 g (7 oz) greek yoghurt or *soy yoghurt

TOPPING

berries or fruit of choice

1   Preheat the oven to 180°C (350°F/Gas 4). Line a baking tray with parchment paper.

2   For the granola, mash up the bananas in a bowl with a fork and add the maple syrup, coconut oil, vanilla seeds and salt. In another bowl mix together the remaining dry ingredients and add to the wet mixture. Stir until well combined. Spread out on the baking sheet and bake for about 20–25 minutes until golden brown. Make sure to stir it from time to time so that the granola is evenly baked. Take out of the oven and leave to cool completely.

3   Meanwhile, make the rhubarb compote. Cut the rhubarb and peaches into small pieces. Put the chopped fruit into a saucepan together with the water and lemon juice. Cook over a medium heat for about 15 minutes until the fruits are softened. Pour into a bowl and stir in the vanilla extract and 2 teaspoons of the maple syrup.

4   In a separate bowl, mix the yoghurt with the remaining maple syrup and add a dash of lemon juice if desired.

5   Spoon some rhubarb compote into glasses, followed by a spoonful of yoghurt, then some granola, and repeat this layering right to the top. Sprinkle some granola on top and garnish with your chosen fruit.

GRANOLA   You can store the granola in an airtight jar for up to 2 weeks.

RED RHUBARB   Red rhubarb doesn't need to be peeled. It's a lot milder and less bitter in the taste compared to green rhubarb.

Sweet Toast Three Ways

Easy to make, versatile and tasty.
Whenever you're in a hurry in the morning but still want to eat something filling and
nutritious without losing too much time, these toasts are exactly what you're looking for.
The choice of bread is yours, simply make sure it's wholewheat and has no added sugar.
To make a lighter version, replace the bread with brown rice cakes
or wholewheat crackers.

SERVES 1 / RSF

3 slices wholewheat bread or brown rice
cakes

ALMOND & RASPBERRY

2–3 teaspoons almond butter

2 teaspoons sugar-free or home-made
berry jam (see page 76)

1 tablespoon raspberries

GREEK YOGHURT & HONEY

1 tablespoon Greek yoghurt

2 teaspoons honey

2–3 teaspoons crushed pistachios

1 tablespoon blueberries

PEANUT BUTTER & BANANA

2–3 teaspoons peanut butter

1 teaspoon honey

½ ripe banana

2–3 teaspoons crushed nuts of choice

1   If you use bread for the base, toast the slices until golden
brown and lay them out on a kitchen board.

2   Spread each slice of toast or rice cake with the nut
butter or yoghurt. Then drizzle over the jam or honey, and
sprinkle the different fruits and nuts on top.

TIP   Two of these toasts are perfect for a simple, quick and
nutritious breakfast. If you are really hungry, three toasts
should be enough! As a snack one toast is ample. Let your
creativity run wild – try out new combinations and find out
what you like best.

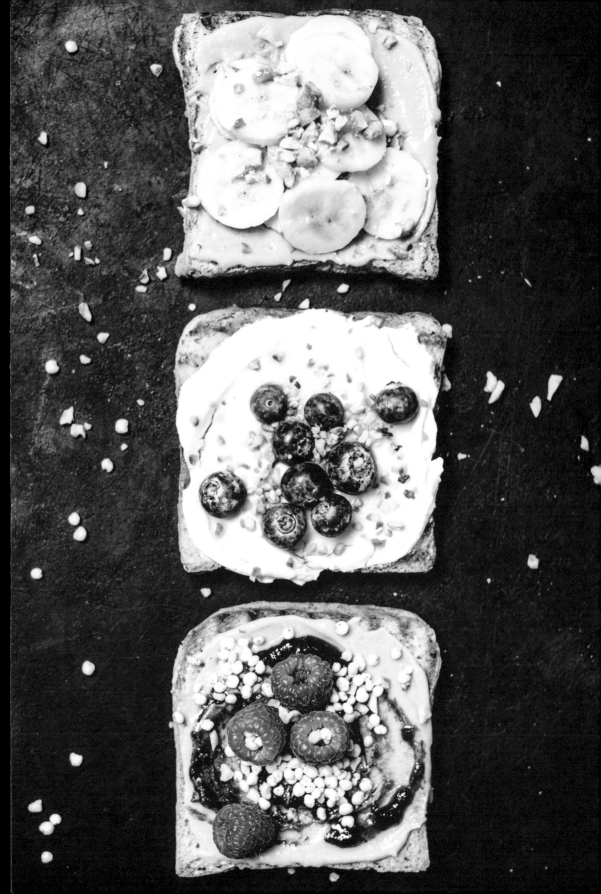

Baked Berries Topped with Oat & Cornflake Crumble

A recipe for every season.

Baked berries topped with this irresistible and crunchy crumble will make you melt,
I promise! It's perfect to enjoy on a cold autumn or winter morning and warms you up
from the inside. I'm sure that crumble is something we all love, but it usually contains a
lot of sugar and butter. This oat and cornflake crumble is completely guilt-free and its
crunch and flavour make it so delicious. Using rice syrup to sweeten it will
guarantee you even more crunchiness. To all the crumble fans, try this recipe.
It's so easy I guarantee you will fall in love with it right away.

SERVES 2 / DF, VGN, RSF

CRUMBLE

3 tablespoons oats (oatmeal)

3 tablespoons sugar-free cornflakes

1 tablespoon coconut oil, melted

1 tablespoon almond butter

2–3 teaspoons rice syrup or sweetener
of choice

1 teaspoon vanilla extract

FILLING

250 g (9 oz/2 cups) fresh or frozen mixed
berries

1 tablespoon coconut sugar or sweetener of
choice, e.g. maple syrup

TOPPINGS

fresh figs

berries of choice

1   Preheat the oven to 180°C (350°F/Gas 4).

2   To make the crumble, put the oats and cornflakes into
a bowl and crumble them with your hands. Add the coconut
oil, almond butter, rice syrup and vanilla extract and stir
until well combined.

3   For the filling, put the berries into a baking dish (about
10 × 20 cm/4 × 8 in), sprinkle coconut sugar on top, give it
a quick stir and equally distribute the crumble on top. Cut
the figs into quarters and place on top of the crumble.

4   Place the crumble on the middle shelf of the oven and
bake for about 20 minutes until golden brown.

5   Remove the baking dish from the oven, let it cool for a
few minutes so that the crumble gets crunchy and serve
warm with some fresh berries.

TIP   If you want to serve this crumble as a dessert, have a
scoop or two of banana ice cream with it. For breakfast, you
can add some yoghurt of your choice sweetened with a
little honey – both options taste great.

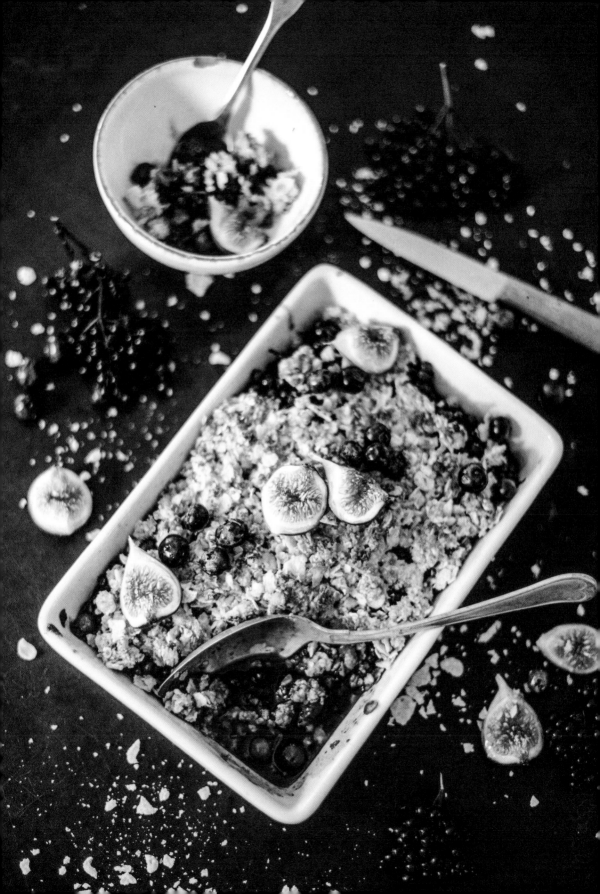

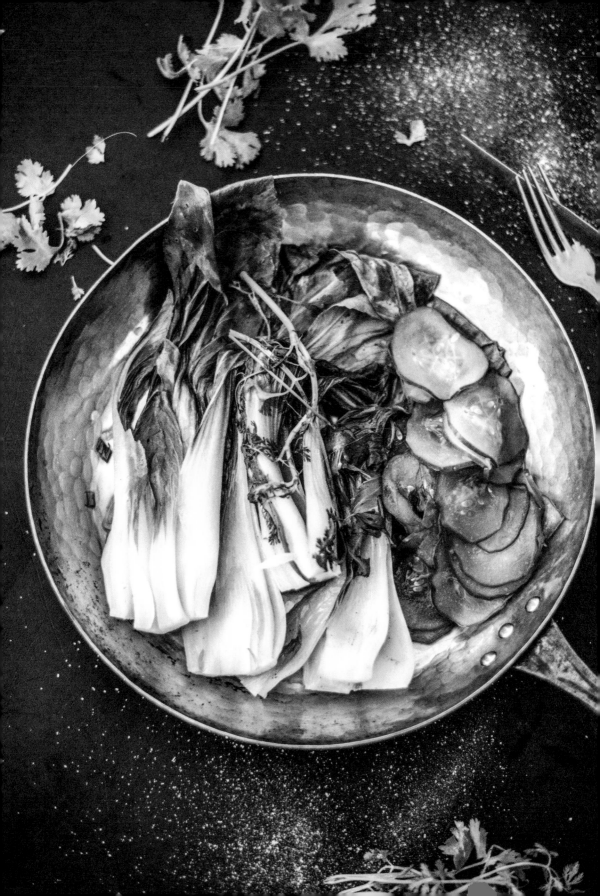

MAIN DISHES & SNACKS

Perfect to fill you up!

GF= GLUTEN-FREE · DF= DAIRY-FREE
V= VEGETARIAN · VGN= VEGAN · RSF= REFINED-SUGAR-FREE

Home-made Spelt Tagliatelle with Mediterranean Vegetables

Simply imagine the Italian scenery and the food will do the rest.

If there's something I personally won't and can't say no to, it has to be home-made pasta. What's better than a good plate of home-made pasta with fresh veggies, a drizzle of extra virgin olive oil and some creamy ricotta? Not much, I'd say. And that's exactly why this recipe is in this book, for you to try and experience the same. Close your eyes while eating, imagine the beautiful scenery of Italy in front of you. There is no reason to fly all the way to Italy when you can easily have your special Italian experience in the comfort of your own home.

SERVES 3-4 / V, RSF

PASTA DOUGH

300 g (10½ oz) wholemeal spelt flour, plus extra for dusting

1 teaspoon sea salt

2 large eggs (room temperature)

2 tablespoons extra virgin olive oil

4–6 tablespoons water

VEGETABLES

1 large aubergine (eggplant), cut into 5 mm (¼ in) thick slices

2 courgettes (zucchinis), cut into 5 mm (¼ in) thick slices

20–24 cherry tomatoes, halved

salt and freshly ground black pepper

1 teaspoon onion powder

2 garlic cloves

2 tablespoons extra virgin olive oil

1 tablespoon basil leaves, chopped

4 handfuls of spinach

150–200 g (5–7 oz) ricotta

few whole basil leaves, to serve

drizzle of lemon juice, to serve

drizzle of honey, to serve

1   For the pasta dough, mix the flour with the salt, sift it onto the work surface and make a well in the centre. Crack the eggs into a glass and mix with the oil and 3 tablespoons of water, then pour into the well. Stir together with a fork.

2   Knead the dough for 8–10 minutes until soft and smooth. Depending on the consistency you might have to add some more water. Form it into a ball and let it stand at room temperature underneath a bowl for 40–50 minutes.

3   Preheat the oven to 160°C (320°F/Gas 3) and line a baking tray with with parchment paper.

4   Lay out the vegetables on the prepared baking tray. Season with salt and pepper, onion powder and garlic. Drizzle the olive oil on top, basil on top and roast for 30-40 minutes.

5   Cut the pasta dough in half. Sprinkle some spelt flour onto the work surface and roll out the dough very thinly. Fold in half again, dust the work surface with more flour, then roll out once more. Cut into 1.5 cm (½ in) wide strips.

6   Bring a large saucepan of salted water to the boil and add the tagliatelle. Cook for 3–5 minutes until it floats to the top. Drain, then return the pasta to the pan with a drizzle of olive oil. Add the roasted vegetables, spinach, ricotta, basil lemon juice and honey to the pasta. Serve with extra ricotta.

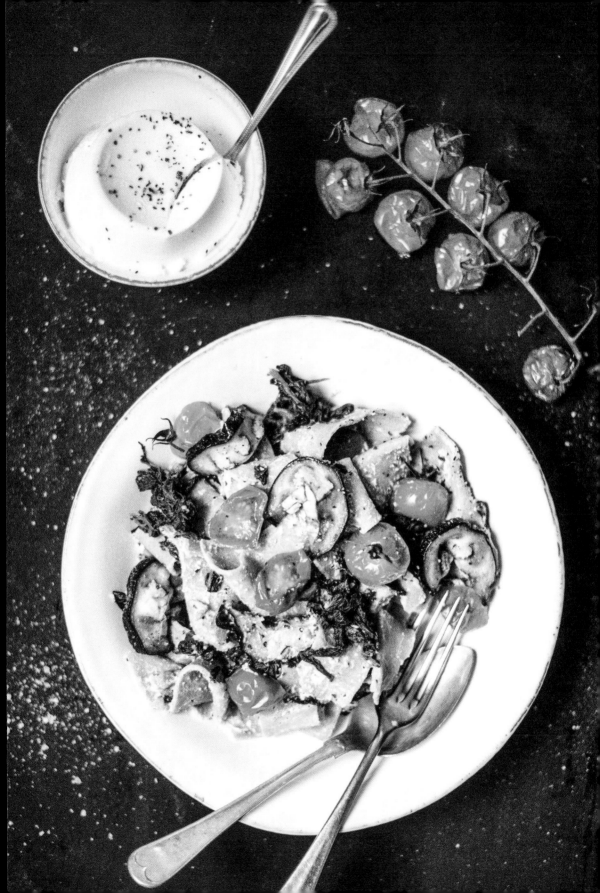

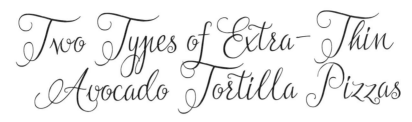

Two Types of Extra-Thin Avocado Tortilla Pizzas

Who's ready for a new kind of pizza?

This wholewheat tortilla pizza is a great alternative to the traditional Italian pizza.
It's really easy to make, and so healthy and nourishing. Although you're not biting into a
cheesy pizza, this delicious alternative gives you the same feeling. And besides that, this
is a completely new taste experience. The avocado, as one of the main ingredients, brings
creaminess and provides healthy fats. This pizza is ready in only
ten minutes and can be served as a main meal or starter.

————————————— SERVES 2 / RSF —————————————

AVOCADO & COURGETTE PIZZA

1 wholewheat tortilla

1 ripe avocado

2 tablespoons cottage cheese or soy yoghurt

1 teaspoon honey, plus extra to serve

salt and freshly ground black pepper

½ teaspoon paprika

1 courgette (zucchini)

1–2 teaspoons olive oil

goat's cheese or grated Parmesan, to serve

AVOCADO & SALMON PIZZA

1 wholewheat tortilla

1 ripe avocado

2 tablespoons low-fat cream cheese

1 teaspoon onion powder

1 teaspoon garlic powder

salt and freshly ground black pepper

2–3 teaspoons lemon juice

150–200 g (5–7 oz) salmon

dill, to serve

AVOCADO & COURGETTE PIZZA

1   Mash together the avocado, cottage cheese, honey, a pinch
of salt and pepper and the paprika. Spread onto the tortilla.

2   Cut the courgette into slices, drizzle over the olive oil and
season with salt and pepper. Griddle or fry the courgettes
until you can see the grill marks or they are golden brown.

3   Heat up a large frying pan (skillet), add the tortilla and
fry over a medium heat for about 5 minutes until the tortilla
has darkened a bit. Take off the heat and put onto a plate.

4   Top with the courgettes, drizzle with some honey if
desired, and add some goat's cheese for extra creaminess
or some grated Parmesan. Garnish with fresh herbs and cut
into slices.

AVOCADO & SALMON PIZZA

1   Mash up half of the avocado with the cream cheese, onion
and garlic powders, salt and pepper and 1–2 teaspoons of the
lemon juice until well combined. Spread onto the tortilla.

2   Heat up a large frying pan, add the tortilla and fry over
a medium heat for about 5 minutes until the tortilla has
darkened a bit. Take off the heat and put onto a plate.

3   Dice the other half of the avocado, season with salt and
pepper, and scatter over the tortilla.

4   Tear the salmon into smaller pieces and add on top of
the tortilla. Sprinkle some dill and 1 teaspoon of lemon juice
over the tortilla and cut into slices.

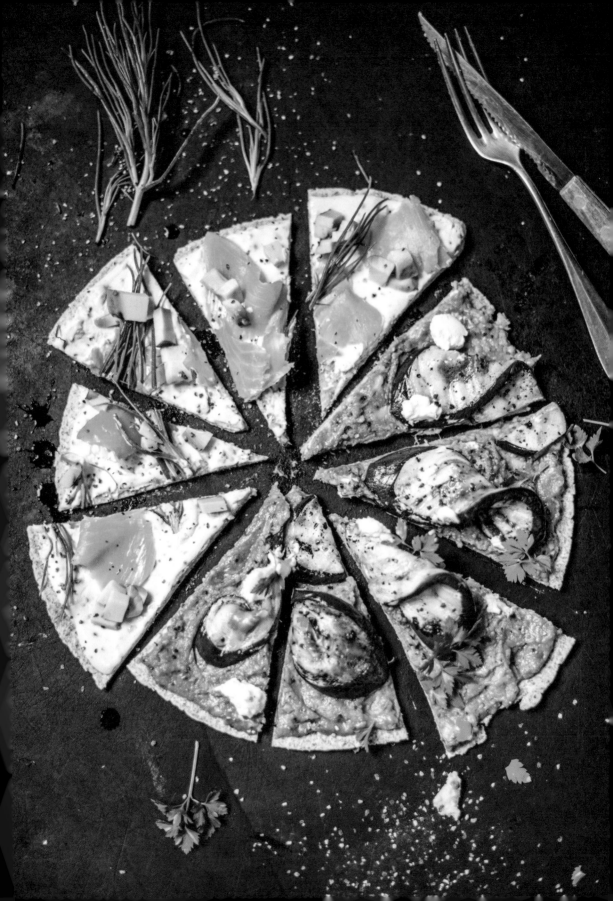

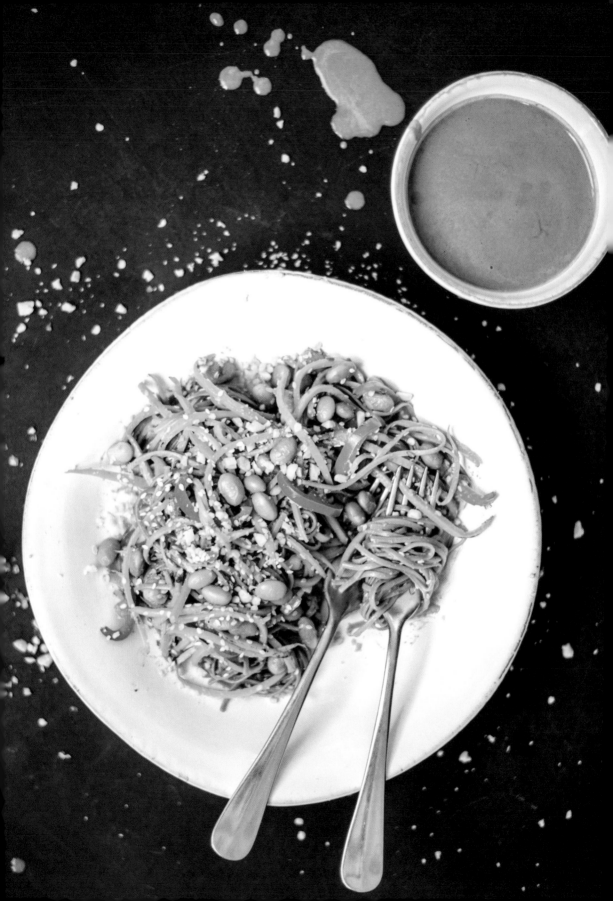

Brown Rice Noodles with Crispy Vegetables & Peanut Soy Sauce

This sauce gives the noodles the right kick.

When I invite friends over for dinner, I love to make this noodle dish. The combination of sweet, salty and spicy makes it a real taste experience. The brown rice noodles are a great alternative to the white rice noodles or egg noodles used in most Asian dishes, because they are made out of 100 percent brown rice. Together with the crispy fried vegetables and the peanut soy sauce – that I could eat on its own, by the way – you have an incredibly tasty and filling dish ready in no time.

SERVES 2 / DF, GF*, V, VGN, RSF

160–180 g (5½–6½ oz) brown rice noodles

crushed peanuts, to serve

VEGETABLES

1 teaspoon coconut oil

4 tablespoons edamame

2 carrots

1 red (bell) pepper

1 tablespoon sesame seeds

1 tablespoon crushed peanuts

PEANUT SOY SAUCE

2 tablespoons peanut butter

2–3 tablespoons *tamari or soy sauce

4 tablespoons milk of choice, e.g. soy, almond, rice milk

2–3 teaspoons maple syrup or sweetener of choice

½–1 teaspoon chilli powder

2 teaspoons onion powder

2 teaspoons garlic powder

salt and freshly ground black pepper

1   Bring a large saucepan of salted water to the boil. Add the brown rice noodles, bring back to the boil, then reduce the heat to medium. Cook for 5–6 minutes, drain, rinse with cold water and set aside.

2   For the vegetables, cut the pepper and carrots into thin slices. Heat up the coconut oil in a frying pan, add the edamame, carrot and pepper slices and fry for 5–6 minutes. Add the sesame seeds and crushed peanuts, lower the heat and let it cook for another 2-3 minutes, stirring from time to time. Take off the heat when they still have a slight crunch.

3   In the meantime, prepare the peanut soy sauce by blending all the ingredients into a smooth and creamy sauce.

4   Add the noodles and sauce to the fried vegetables, heat up again and stir until well combined.

5   Serve topped with some crushed peanuts.

VARIATIONS   I personally love to drizzle some honey on top at the very end. The sweet taste goes so well with this dish. Also, for those of you who like it spicy like me, add some extra chilli or put Sriracha on the table when serving.

Black Rice Paella with Shiitake & Wheatgrass Aioli

Yum, yum and yum, yum, yum!

One spring I took a trip to Barcelona where, among other things, I kept a look out for healthy, organic restaurants that have a similar cooking style and use similar ingredients to me. I discovered a beautiful, modern and rustic restaurant in a small back street in the old part of the city – exactly what I was looking for. It was really hard to choose something from their amazing menu but I decided on a paella made with black rice. I didn't really know exactly what was in it, but I tried creating something similar. Here's my version, which will hopefully convince every Spanish paella lover as well. A must try!

———— SERVES 2-3 / GF, DF*, V, VGN* ————

PAELLA

1 tablespoon olive oil

1 onion, chopped

1 garlic clove, chopped

250 g (9 oz) black rice

100 ml (3½ fl oz) white wine

800 ml (27 fl oz) vegetable stock (broth)

250 ml (8½ fl oz) coconut milk

200 g (7 oz) shiitake mushrooms

1 small broccoli

4–5 tablespoons fresh or frozen and thawed edamame

fresh thyme

WHEATGRASS AIOLI

½ ripe avocado

100 g (3½ oz) *soy yoghurt or Greek yoghurt

zest and juice of 1 lime

salt and freshly ground black pepper

1 teaspoon onion powder

1 garlic clove, chopped, or 2 teaspoons garlic powder

1 teaspoon almond butter

2–3 tablespoons wheatgrass powder

drizzle of olive oil

1–2 teaspoons maple syrup or sweetener of choice

fresh thyme, to serve

1   For the paella, heat up the olive oil in a frying pan, add the chopped onion and garlic and sauté for a few minutes. Add the black rice, stir well, then pour in the white wine. Cook over a high heat for a few more minutes while gradually stirring in the vegetable stock.

2   Pour in the coconut milk, stir well and cook over a medium–low heat for about 1 hour. Stir from time to time.

3   Slice the shiitake mushrooms. Cut the stem off the broccoli, tear it into florets and cut them into slices.

4   Add the mushrooms, broccoli and edamame to the rice, add some thyme, stir well and continue cooking until the rice is cooked.

5   For the aioli, blend all the ingredients except the thyme to a creamy and smooth consistency. Garnish with fresh thyme and cool in the fridge until the rice is ready.

6   Add a splash of coconut milk to the rice and stir again. Spoon onto plates and top with the aioli.

WHEATGRASS   This superfood is available in powdered form either online or at almost every health food store. Wheatgrass is extremely rich in minerals and vitamins, and has a distinctively delicious taste. You can add a teaspoon of wheatgrass to your daily breakfast as well or even make a wheatgrass soy vanilla latte.

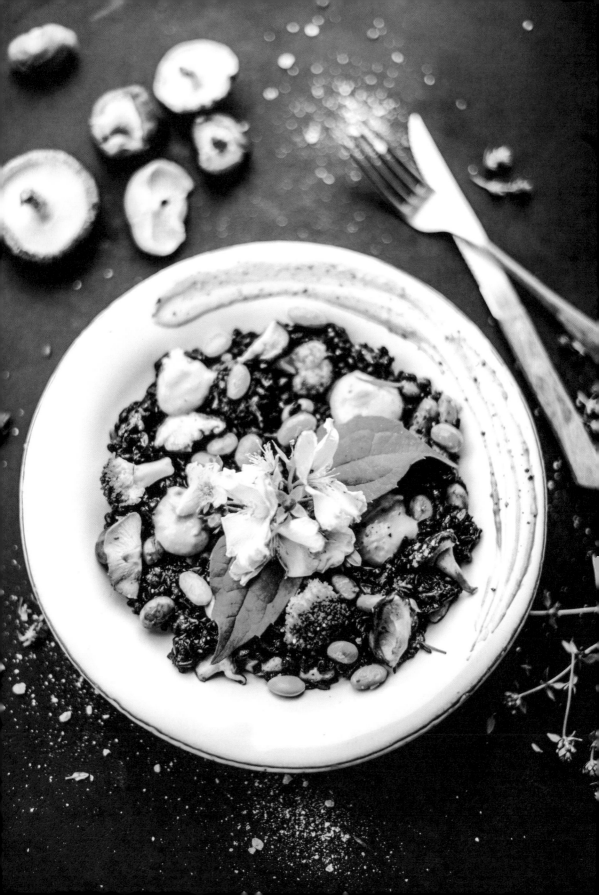

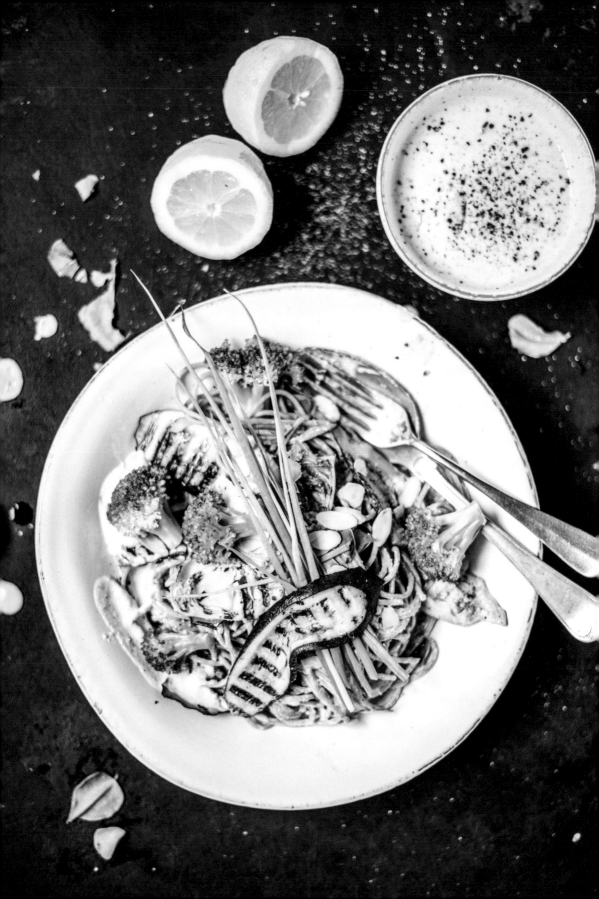

Wholewheat Spaghetti with Lemony Goat's Cheese Sauce

If you like goat's cheese and spaghetti, this dish is made just for you. Being Swiss and growing up with cheese, I prefer full-fat over low-fat, but you can also use low-fat goat's cheese for this recipe. The lemon balances out the different flavours really well and gives this spaghetti dish, together with the grilled vegetables, a fresh taste.

SERVES 4–5 / V, RSF

400 g (14 oz) wholewheat spaghetti

4 tablespoons flaked (slivered) almonds, roasted

lemon juice, to serve

fresh chives, to garnish

FOR THE VEGETABLES

2 courgettes (zucchini)

10–14 artichoke hearts in salted water

2 teaspoons lemon juice

1 tablespoon olive oil

salt and freshly ground black pepper

1 teaspoon onion powder

1 large broccoli

1 teaspoon vegetable stock (broth) powder or 1 stock cube

GOAT'S CHEESE SAUCE

4 tablespoons fresh goat's cheese

zest and juice of 1 lemon

2 teaspoons garlic powder

½ teaspoon sea salt

½ teaspoon ground pepper

1 teaspoon maple syrup or sweetener of choice

250–300 ml (8½–10 fl oz) milk of choice, e.g. soy, almond, rice milk

1 spring onion (scallion), chopped

bunch of fresh chives, chopped

6–8 kaffir lime leaves, crumbled

1   Heat up a griddle pan or preheat the oven to 180°C (350°F/Gas 4).

2   Slice the courgettes diagonally and drain and quarter the artichoke hearts. Season the vegetables with salt, pepper and onion powder, and drizzle the olive oil and lemon juice on top.

3   Place the vegetables onto the griddle and cook until you can see the grill marks. If you don't have a griddle pan, spread out the vegetables in a single layer on the baking tray and roast in the oven for about 20 minutes.

4   Make up the stock according to the packet instructions. Cut the stem off the broccoli and tear it into florets. Cook in the stock for 3–4 minutes so that the broccoli keeps a slight crunch.

5   Bring a large saucepan of salted water to the boil, add the spaghetti and cook until al dente.

6   While the spaghetti is cooking, prepare the goat's cheese sauce. Add the cheese, lemon, garlic powder, salt and pepper, maple syrup and milk to a saucepan over a medium heat. Cook for 5–6 minutes, reduce the heat and add the spring onion, chives and kaffir lime leaves. Stir again and turn off the heat.

7   Put the almonds into a dry frying pan (skillet) and toast over a medium heat until golden brown. Take off the heat and let them cool completely.

8   Drain the spaghetti, transfer it back into the pan and pour the sauce over the pasta. Stir well over a medium heat for 1–2 minutes. Serve into bowls, top with the vegetables and roasted almond slices and if desired, add another splash of lemon juice for some extra freshness. Garnish with chives.

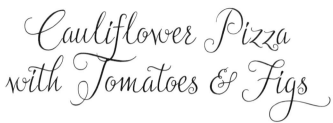

Cauliflower Pizza with Tomatoes & Figs

The real pizza feeling with a flourless dough.

A pizza dough without flour in it at all – how is this possible? By making the dough out of cauliflower! It might sound a little bit weird to you at first, but wait until you've tried it. The cauliflower base is an amazing option for you to make when you don't want to eat carbs but still want to eat a nourishing pizza that keeps you full and satisfied. This pizza is not only delicious right out of the oven, but also served in slices as a starter or as a snack on a night with friends.

—————— 1 PIZZA/SERVES 1-2 (26–28 CM/10–11 IN) / GF, V, RSF ——————

CAULIFLOWER BASE

350 g (12 oz) cauliflower
salt and freshly ground black pepper
1 teaspoon onion powder
1 teaspoon garlic powder
60–80 g (2–3 oz) Parmesan, grated
10–15 basil leaves
1 teaspoon chilli powder (optional)
1 egg, whisked

TOPPINGS

3 ripe tomatoes
handful of cherry tomatoes
2 fresh figs
1½–2 tablespoons olive oil
grated Parmesan, to serve
fresh basil leaves, to serve
1 tablespoon balsamic cream, to serve

1   Preheat the oven to 220°C (430°F/Gas 7).

2   To make the pizza base, grate the cauliflower, add a pinch of salt, put it onto kitchen paper and squeeze out the excess liquid. Put the grated cauliflower into a bowl and add the onion powder, garlic powder, grated Parmesan and basil. Season with some more salt and pepper, if desired, and add the chilli if you want some spice. Pour in the egg and mix everything really well, then form the mixture into a ball with your hands.

3   Line a baking tray with parchment paper and put the cauliflower 'dough' on top. Cover with another piece of parchment paper and roll out the dough to an approximately 5 mm (¼ in) thick circle. Take off the top piece of parchment paper and bake the base on the lower shelf of the oven for 30–40 minutes.

4   Take the cauliflower base out of the oven and prepare the toppings. Cut the tomatoes into slices, halve the cherry tomatoes and quarter the figs and spread everything out onto the base. Drizzle the olive oil on top and bake for another 10–15 minutes.

5   A few minutes before taking the pizza out of the oven, add some grated Parmesan on top to melt. Take the pizza out, garnish with basil leaves, drizzle the balsamic cream on top and cut into slices. Serve right away or cool in the fridge to serve later as an appetiser.

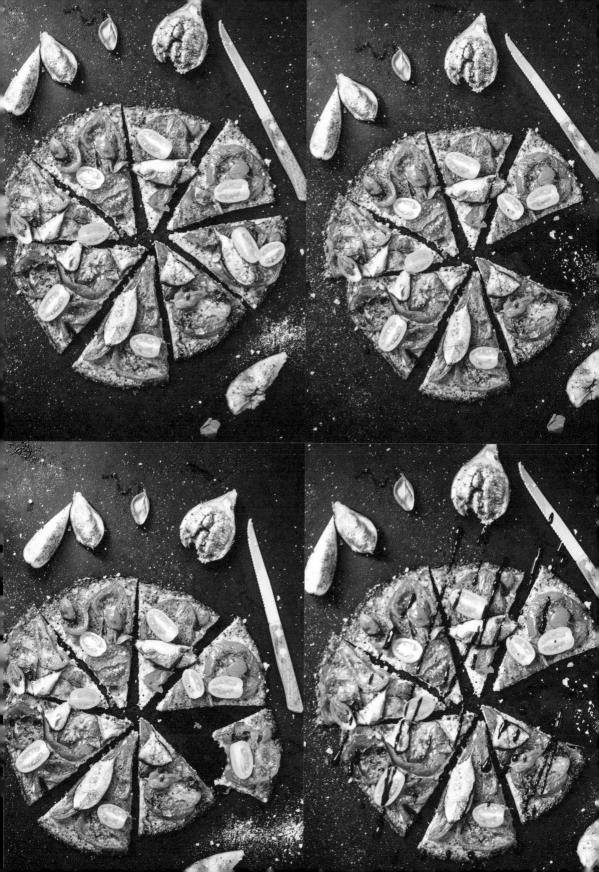

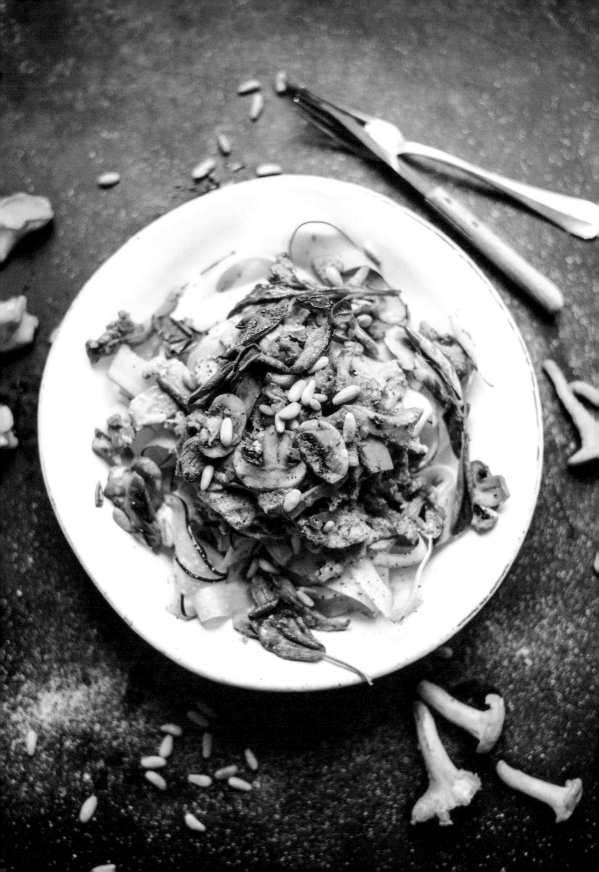

Courgette Tagliatelle & Creamy Mushroom Sauce

On your marks, get set, mushrooms!

I pretty much love every type of mushroom and could eat them every day. Most of you probably know pasta in combination with mushrooms only with a creamy, fatty sauce. The sauce in this recipe doesn't contain any cream or oil at all; it's only made with soy milk products but it's still very smooth and creamy, not to mention tasty. It's important to mix the sauce well with the courgette tagliatelle in order to get the full flavour.

SERVES 2-3 / (GF), DF, V, VGN, RSF

TAGLIATELLE

3–4 large courgettes (zucchini)

vegetable stock (broth) powder

MUSHROOM-SAUCE

80 g (3 oz) pine nuts

300 g (10½ oz) soy yoghurt

1 tablespoon lemon juice

1 teaspoon onion powder

1 teaspoon garlic powder

1–2 teaspoons maple syrup or sweetener of choice

500 g (1 lb 2 oz) button mushrooms

100 g (3½ oz) ceps

300 g (10½ oz) chanterelles

2 teaspoons coconut oil

1 large onion, chopped

1 garlic clove, chopped

salt and freshly ground black pepper

½ teaspoon chilli powder

splash of soy milk

1 tablespoon pine nuts, roasted

grated Parmesan, to serve

1   For the sauce, toast the pine nuts in a dry frying pan (skillet) over a medium heat until golden brown. Pour over some boiling water, take off the heat and leave the nuts to swell for about 10 minutes. Drain and add the pine nuts into a blender along with the yoghurt, lemon juice, onion powder, garlic powder and maple syrup. Blend for about 4–5 minutes to a smooth and creamy consistency.

2   Wash the mushrooms and dry them off with a towel. Slice the button mushrooms and quarter the chanterelles. Heat up the coconut oil in a large frying pan (skillet), add the onion and garlic, and fry until shiny and golden brown. Add the mushrooms and fry over a high heat, stirring constantly. Season with salt, pepper and chilli powder, turn down the heat and let it cook for a few more minutes. Add the pine nut sauce to the mushrooms, stir well and leave on a low heat. Add a dash of soy milk if the sauce gets too thick.

3   For the courgette tagliatelle, wash and halve the courgettes, remove the soft core and use a vegetable peeler or spiralizer to peel into ribbons.

4   Heat up 100 ml (3½ fl oz) of water in a large pan, add the vegetable stock, then add the courgette ribbons and cook for 1–2 minutes so that they soften a little bit but still retain their crunch.

5   Drain the courgettes, add them to the mushroom sauce and stir until well combined. Serve on plates and sprinkle some grated Parmesan on top. Garnish with roasted pine nuts and enjoy.

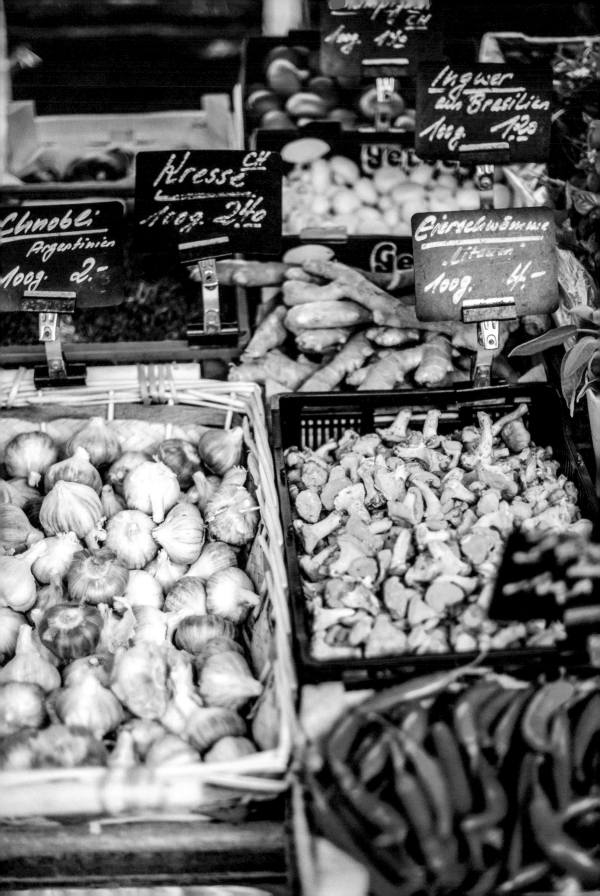

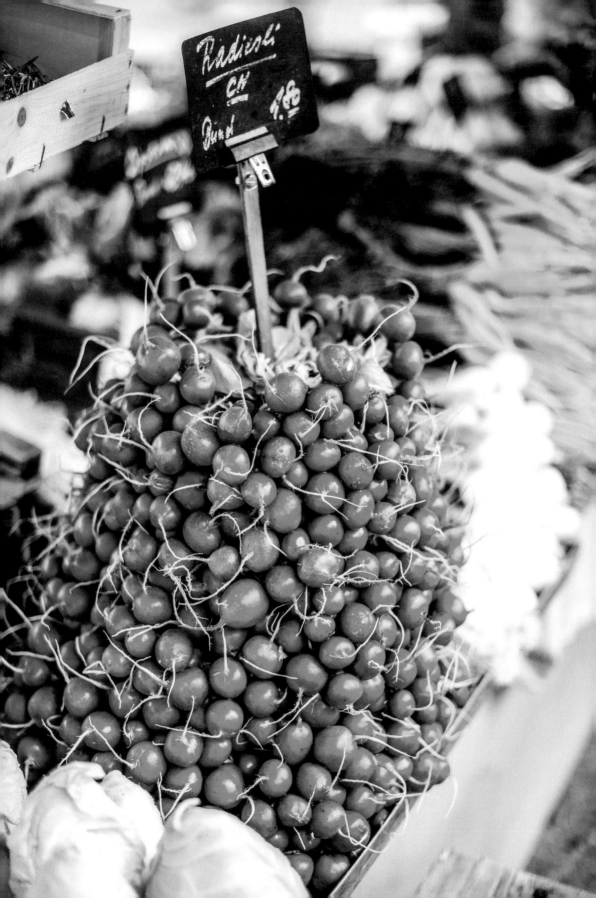

Fusilli with Kale & Mint Pesto

Aroma and taste: irresistible times two.

I can remember the first bite of this pasta perfectly! I was totally blown away and found myself in a completely new world of flavour. The pesto is a real taste explosion. Store-bought pesto contains a lot of oil and cheese. I don't use cheese at all and only add a little bit of olive oil. To make the pesto lighter and creamier I add cashews and some yoghurt at the end. Instead of normal pasta I use wholewheat spelt fusilli. Wholewheat products support a healthy diet and are better for your digestive system.

———————————— SERVES 3-4 / V, RSF ————————————

PESTO

200 g (7 oz) kale

4 sprigs of mint (approx. 30 leaves)

1–2 garlic cloves

1 teaspoon onion powder

1 tablespoon lemon juice

50 g (2 oz) cashews

1 teaspoon maple syrup or sweetener of choice

1 tablespoon olive oil

salt and freshly ground black pepper

6–8 tablespoons yoghurt

PASTA & VEGETABLES

400 g (14 oz) wholewheat fusilli

handful of okra

1 teaspoon coconut oil or olive oil

mint leaves

200 g (7 oz) spinach or kale

salt and freshly ground black pepper

crushed cashews

1   For the pesto, put the kale, mint, garlic, onion powder, lemon juice, cashews, maple syrup and olive oil into a food processor and blend for 1–2 minutes. The mixture shouldn't be too smooth and should still have some small herby pieces in it. Season and add the yoghurt, then stir well and set aside.

2   Bring a large saucepan of salted water to the boil, add the fusilli and cook until al dente.

3   Meanwhile, heat up the olive oil in a frying pan (skillet) over a high heat and fry the okra for a few minutes until they have softened. Add a splash of water, turn down the heat to medium and add the mint leaves and spinach or kale. Season and cook over a medium–low heat for 5–6 minutes.

4   Drain the fusilli, put it back into the pan and add the vegetables to the pasta. Stir well.

5   Serve onto plates, top with the pesto and garnish with crushed cashews. To get the maximum taste, add the pesto to the fusilli along with the vegetables, heat up again very quickly and stir until well combined.

VARIATION   You can also add about a third of the pesto to the fusilli and put the rest of the pesto on the table for those who would like to add a little more to their pasta.

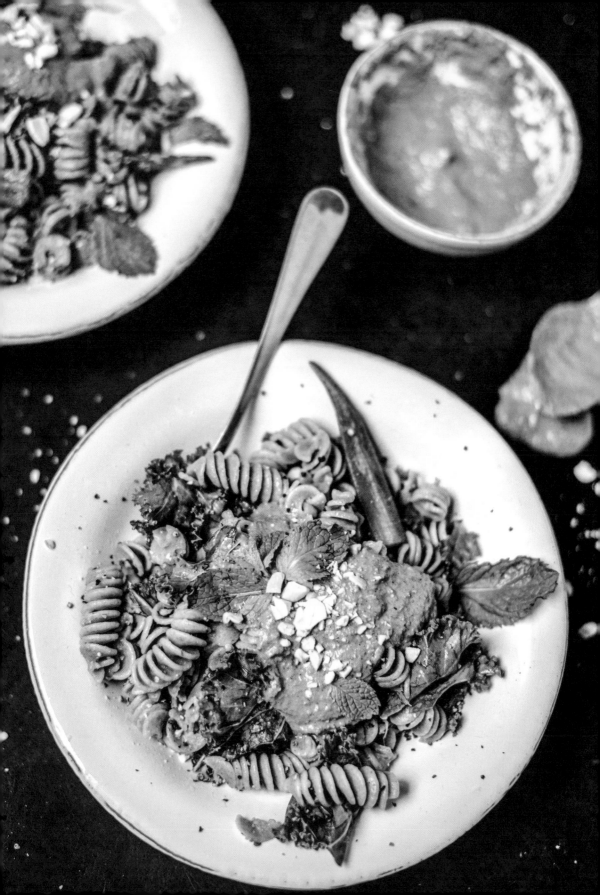

Zoodles with Dreamy Creamy Pumpkin Bolognese

How to make eating pasta more fun.

It's really hard to say no to a plate of white pasta with a good bolognese. If you say no, it's probably because you don't want to eat a heavy dish or because you don't want to eat refined carbohydrates. Courgette noodles, also called zoodles, promise a light but filling, delicious dish that's low in calories. The noodles consist of fresh courgettes only. They're either spiralized or are cut into long and thin slices with a julienne peeler. Because the courgette is pretty neutral in taste, a good and well-spiced sauce is a must! This is a dish that you can enjoy completely-guilt free, have a large portion of and still have the 'I'm eating spaghetti bolognese' feeling.

SERVES 3-4 / GF, V*, VGN*

BOLOGNESE

1 tablespoon olive oil

1 small onion, chopped

2 garlic cloves, chopped

400 g (14 oz) minced (ground) beef or *soy meat/vegetables of choice

1 teaspoon paprika

salt and freshly ground black pepper

200 ml (7 fl oz) red wine

4 large tomatoes, diced

200 g (7 oz) tomato purée (paste)

350 g (12 oz) pumpkin, peeled and diced

bunch of parsley, chopped

chilli powder (optional)

100 g (3½ oz) grated Parmesan or *vegan Parmesan/cashew cheese

ZOODLES

4–5 courgettes (zucchinis)

300–400 g (10½–14 oz) kale, sliced

1 teaspoon vegetable stock (broth) powder

1   For the bolognese, heat up the olive oil in a frying pan (skillet), add the onion and garlic and fry until golden brown. Add the minced beef, stir, season with paprika, salt and pepper, and stir for 1–2 more minutes. Pour in the red wine, bring to the boil and lower the heat.

2   Add the tomatoes, tomato purée, 100 g (3½ oz) of the pumpkin and the parsley. Cook over a low–medium heat for 25–35 minutes and stir from time to time.

3   In another pan, heat up a good splash of water, add the remaining diced pumpkin and cook until the pumpkin pieces fall apart. Drain, add to a food processor and blend until smooth.

4   In a frying pan (skillet), heat up 100 ml (3½ fl oz) of water with the stock. Cut the courgettes into noodles with a spiralizer or julienne peeler. Steam for 1–2 minutes until they have softened, then take out of the pan, reserving the stock. Don't leave them in the pan for too long – they should keep their crunch!

5   Add the kale to the pan with the remaining vegetable stock and soften for 2–3 minutes. Drain and set aside.

6   Pour the pumpkin purée into the bolognese, stir well and season with salt, pepper and chilli if you like it a little spicy.

7   Tip the zoodles and kale into the bolognese, add half of the Parmesan, stir well and divide onto plates. Top with the remaining Parmesan and serve.

VARIATIONS   For a vegetarian version, replace the beef with soy meat. For a vegan version, again substitute the beef with soy meat and use vegan Parmesan or cashew cheese.

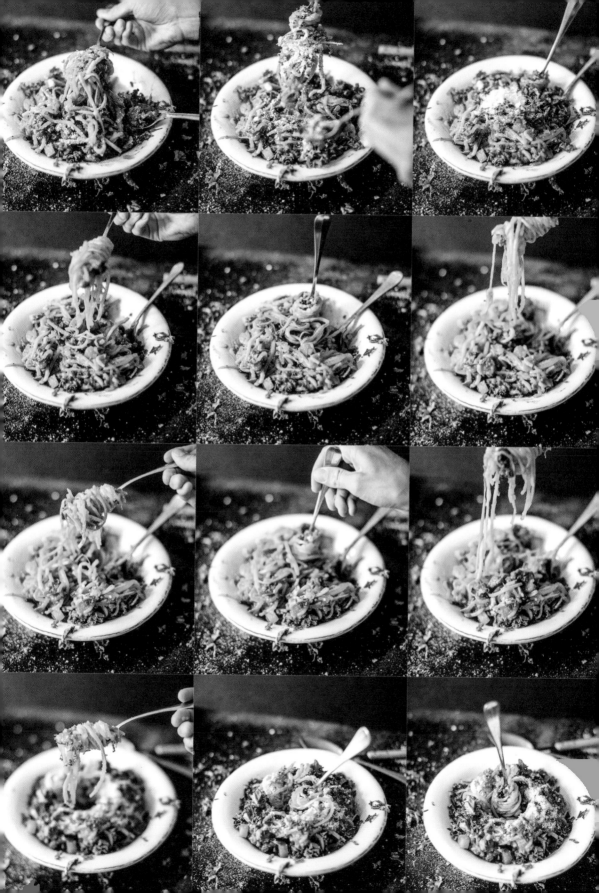

Sweet Potato & Avocado Burger Stacked with Grilled Veggies

Absolutely no need for meat!

Sometimes, a good burger is all you need. But a burger doesn't have to be a bun with a beef patty and a lonely slice of pickle in it. You can create so much taste by combining different ingredients. To me, a mix of grilled or roasted vegetables and fresh vegetables are a must for a good veggie burger. The avocado brings in that creaminess every burger should have and the sweet potato gives a sweet kick. I add some colour with red spinach. Together with a wholewheat sourdough bun, this burger is a real treat.

─────────────── SERVES 2 / DF*, V, VGN*, RSF ───────────────

2 wholewheat sourdough buns

BURGER

1 ripe avocado

½ teaspoon ground paprika

½ teaspoon ground coriander

salt and freshly ground black pepper

1 teaspoon maple syrup or sweetener of choice

2 handfuls of red or green spinach

VEGETABLES

1 sweet potato

1 courgette (zucchini)

1 small aubergine (eggplant)

1–2 tablespoons olive oil

1 tablespoon grated Parmesan or basil pesto or *vegan cheese

salt and freshly ground black pepper

1   Heat up a griddle pan. If you don't have one, heat up the oven to 180°C (350°F/Gas 4) and line a baking tray with parchment paper.

2   For the vegetables, cut the sweet potato into 7 mm (½ in) thick slices. Cut off the ends of the courgette and aubergine and quarter them lengthwise. Put the vegetables into a large bowl, drizzle with olive oil, season, and mix well with your hands. Griddle the vegetables for about 20 minutes until you can see the grill marks or lay them out on parchment paper and roast in the oven for 20–30 minutes.

3   For the burger, put the avocado flesh into a bowl together with the paprika, coriander, salt, pepper and maple syrup. Mash with a fork until well combined.

4   Cut the buns in half and put them onto the griddle or into the oven for a few minutes to crisp up.

5   Transfer the grilled vegetables onto a chopping board. Add the Parmesan or basil pesto to the vegetables and chop everything with a large knife into smaller pieces.

6   Put some spinach on top of the crunchy spelt bun, spread avocado purée on top, add a few slices of the grilled sweet potato and then a large spoonful of the vegetables. Spread the other half of the bun with avocado purée and place on top of the burger.

7   Serve straight away, and don't forget to gobble up everything that falls out of the burger while eating.

TIP   If one burger is not enough for you and you still feel hungry, I suggest to either make the Sweet Potato Fries on page 198 or simply have a salad with home-made dressing on the side.

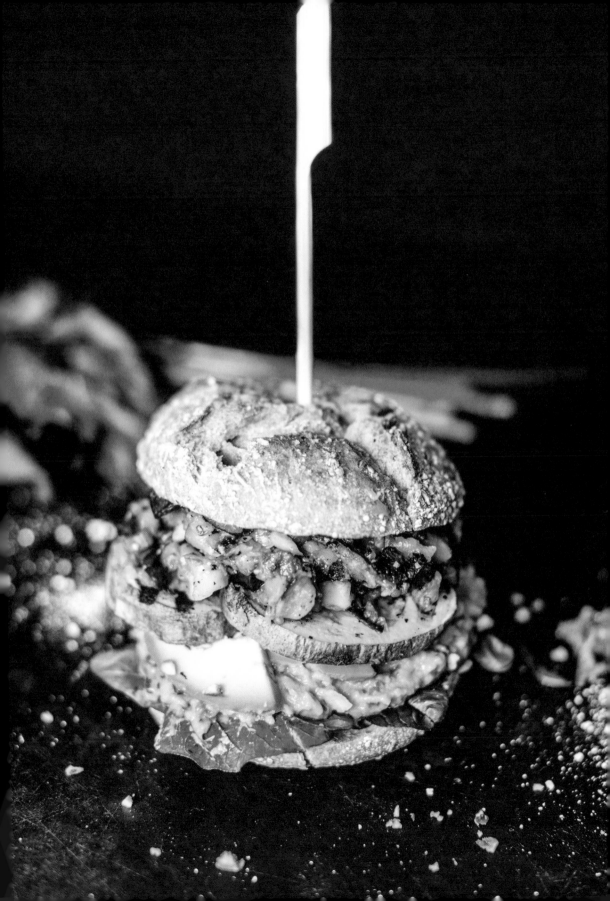

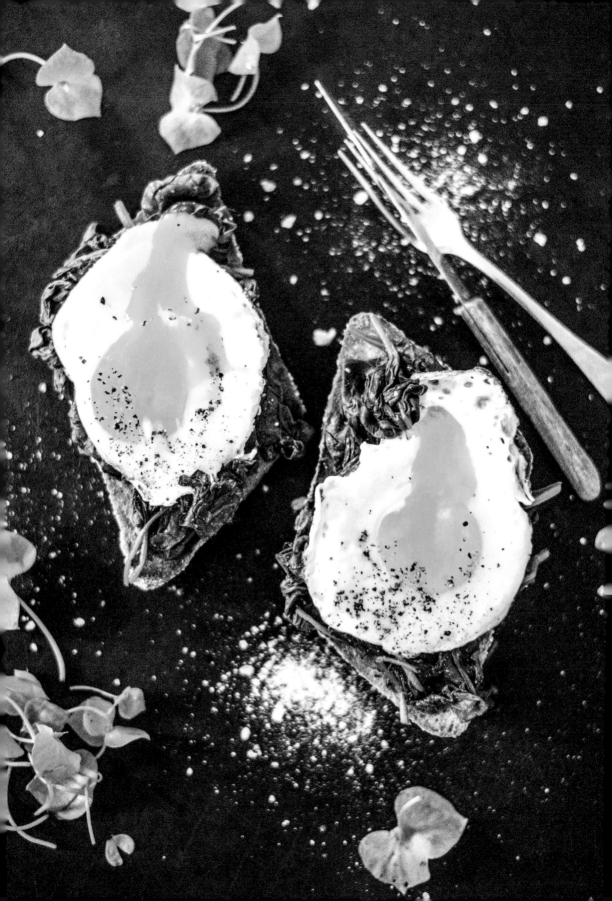

Runny Eggs on Sautéed Spinach & Crispy Wholewheat Bread

Dig in!

'Eat spinach, spinach makes you strong!' Back when I was a kid I used to hear this sentence a lot. And I think kids don't like spinach simply because kids aren't supposed to like spinach, not because of the taste. I'm crazy about spinach — I love including it in my recipes and discovering how versatile it can be with every new recipe. Besides that, it's actually good for you and contains plenty of iron to support our health. Seems like mum and dad were right after all.

SERVES 1 / DF, V, RSF

SPINACH

1 teaspoon vegetable stock (broth) powder

200 g (7 oz) spinach

½ teaspoon garlic powder

½ teaspoon onion powder

BREAD

1 wholewheat bun

1 tablespoon olive oil

EGGS

1–2 teaspoons olive oil or coconut oil

2 large eggs

salt and freshly ground black pepper

1   Heat up a splash of water with the vegetable stock in a frying pan (skillet). Add the spinach, garlic powder and onion powder and sauté for about 2–3 minutes until softened. Take off the heat and drain well.

2   Cut the bun in half, toast until golden brown, then drizzle the olive oil on top. This will give the bread an amazing taste and covers part of your healthy fat intake.

3   Divide the spinach equally on top of the toast.

4   For the eggs, heat up the olive or coconut oil in a frying pan over a medium heat. Crack the eggs one by one into the pan and fry over a low–medium heat for about 5 minutes. Season with salt and pepper and take off the heat while the egg yolk is still runny. Place the eggs on top of the spinach and serve.

TIP   Cut into the runny egg yolk and spread the yolk over the whole bun. So, so good! It's really important to cook the eggs over a low heat so that they cook evenly. Otherwise, the bottom will burn while the top is still raw.

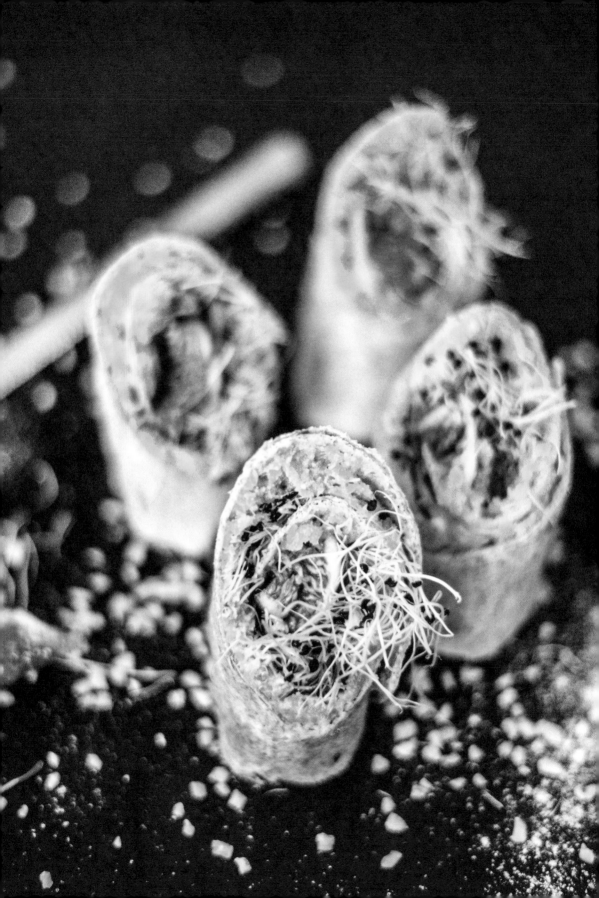

Creamy Cashew Carrot Wraps

The time for boring sandwiches is over – now it's wrap time.
These wraps are so easy to make and just taste incredibly good. The smooth cashew cream
gets a slight crust after frying in the pan that you have to try, because it will almost
knock you down! For some freshness I add some figs as well. We have a huge fig tree
in our garden and I wanted to make this recipe for so long, but I felt like something was
missing. I tried it with fresh and juicy figs and they provide the sweetness that the wrap
needs. Adding onion sprouts gives a good contrast in both the look and taste.

SERVES 2 / DF, V, VGN, RSF

2–3 wholewheat tortillas

CASHEW CREAM

120 g (4 oz) cashews

zest and juice of 1 lemon

150 ml (5 fl oz) milk of choice, e.g. soy, almond, rice milk

1 teaspoon onion powder

1 teaspoon garlic powder

2 teaspoons mild or spicy curry powder

2–3 teaspoons maple syrup or sweetener of choice

salt and freshly ground black pepper

FILLING

6–8 medium sized carrots

50 g (2 oz) onion sprouts

4–5 figs, quartered

1   To make the cashew cream, soak the cashews in hot water for 20–30 minutes. Drain and put into a blender or food processor. Add the remaining ingredients and blend for 4–5 minutes until smooth and creamy. The cream should have quite a thick consistency but you might have to add another splash of milk to make the blending easier.

2   For the filling, peel and grate the carrots. Heat up a dry frying pan (skillet), add the carrots and cashew cream and fry over a medium heat for 3–4 minutes, stirring constantly. Fry for another 3–4 minutes. Reduce the heat. The less you stir now, the better a tasty crust can form.

3   Spread 2–3 tablespoons of the cashew curry carrots on the upper two thirds of each tortilla. Add some fig quarters and onion sprouts on top, fold up the lower part of the wrap and roll in from the side. Halve diagonally and serve as a starter for four people or meal for two.

VARIATION   If you'd like your tortilla to be a little crispy, heat up a frying pan over a medium heat and add the wrap. Fry on all sides until golden brown, take off the heat, let it cool, halve diagonally and serve.

TIP   To save time, soak the cashews overnight or in the morning right after you wake up. There isn't a limit to how long you can soak the cashews for. The longer you do, the creamier the result.

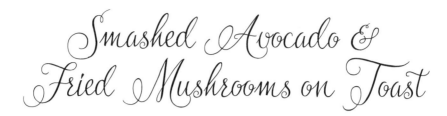

Smashed Avocado & Fried Mushrooms on Toast

An absolute favourite for everyone!
In this recipe, less is definitely more. It's so quick and easy to make.
Whenever I take the first bite of it, I ask myself why I don't make this more often.
Like every day. Twice a day. You can have it for breakfast, brunch, or even for dinner.

SERVES 1 / V, RSF

2 slices wholewheat spelt bread
1 tablespoon pumpkin seeds
lemon juice
cress, to garnish

AVOCADO CREAM
1 small ripe avocado
2 tablespoons cottage cheese
1 teaspoon onion powder
2 teaspoons lemon juice
salt and freshly ground black pepper

MUSHROOMS
1 teaspoon coconut oil
150 g (5 oz) button mushrooms
salt and freshly ground black pepper

1   For the avocado cream, halve the avocado, remove the stone, peel, reserve a quarter of it and put the rest into a bowl. Add the cottage cheese, onion powder and lemon juice to the avocado and mash everything with a fork. Season with salt and pepper to taste.

2   Toast the bread until golden brown in either a toaster or in a frying pan (skillet) over a medium heat.

3   To cook the mushrooms, heat up the coconut oil in a frying pan. Wash the mushrooms, cut them into slices and put them into the pan. Fry for 3–5 minutes, season and take off the heat.

4   Toast the pumpkin seeds in a dry frying pan over a medium heat for a few minutes. Take off the heat and leave to cool.

5   Spread the avocado cream onto the toast and add the fried mushrooms on top. Cut the remaining quarter of the avocado into thin slices and lay on top of the mushrooms. Sprinkle the roasted pumpkin seeds on top, add another splash of lemon juice for some more freshness and garnish with cress.

VARIATIONS   Add a poached egg on top, which provides an extra portion of protein and tastes incredibly good! You can also use different types of bread – simply make sure it doesn't contain white flour, refined sugar or preservatives. For the vegan version, add 1 tablespoon of soy yoghurt instead of the cottage cheese.

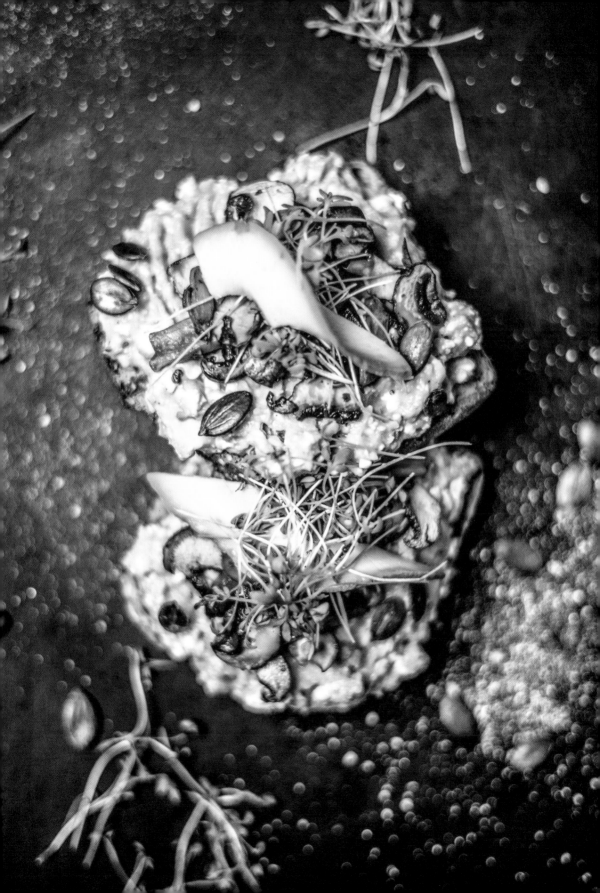

Pulled Chicken Caprese Burger

The classic salad as a burger.

Caprese salad? I'm sure the yumminess bell is ringing in your head right now.
Yes, it's a delicious salad, but it's usually made with plenty of olive oil, full-fat mozzarella
and has way more calories than you would think. I got a little creative with this recipe.
Instead of full-fat mozzarella, I used low-fat mozzarella. I left out the olive oil and white
bread that's usually served with the salad and replaced them with other, more wholesome
ingredients. If that's too much change for you, I promise, the pulled chicken
in this super tasty tomato marinade will make up for it.

───────── SERVES 1 / RSF ─────────

1 wholewheat spelt bun

1 tablespoon tomato purée (paste)

salt and freshly ground black pepper

70–80 g (2½–3 oz) low-fat
  mozzarella

1 large tomato, sliced

basil leaves

lettuce or spinach leaves

PULLED CHICKEN

220–250 g (8–9 oz) chicken breast

1 teaspoon vegetable stock (broth)
  powder

bunch of basil leaves

½ lemon, sliced

3 teaspoons tomato purée (paste)

2 teaspoons honey or sweetener of
  choice

freshly ground black pepper

1 teaspoon paprika

2 teaspoons dried oregano

2 teaspoons balsamic glaze

1 teaspoon onion powder

1 teaspoon garlic powder

1   Preheat the oven to 160°C (320°F/Gas 3).

2   To make the pulled chicken, bring a large saucepan with
200 ml (7 fl oz) of water, the vegetable broth, basil and lemon
slices to the boil. Add the chicken breast, cover with a lid and
cook over a low–medium heat for 12–15 minutes. Take off the
heat but leave the chicken breast in the water for 2–3 more
minutes so that it's well cooked through.

3   Take the chicken out of the pan, drain any excess water,
put it on the work surface and pull into strips with a fork.
Put the pulled chicken into a large bowl, add the remaining
ingredients and mix well. Cover with a towel and set aside. The
chicken will stay juicy and tender in this marinade.

4   Halve the bun and spread the tomato purée over each half.
Season with salt and pepper and add some fresh basil leaves on
top. Tear the mozzarella into pieces and divide it equally between
both halves. Bake in the oven until the mozzarella has melted
(this will take a few minutes longer than with full-fat cheese).
Take out of the oven and add the tomato slices on top.

5   Add some salad on one half, top with the pulled chicken
and place the other half on top. Press down a little, open your
mouth wide, close your eyes and hope that nobody's watching
you eat, because it could get quite messy!

TIP   If you don't want to make a mess or for anything to fall out
of the burger, simply add some pulled chicken on both halves
and eat the halves separately. Problem solved.

VARIATION   If you want the pulled chicken to be hot, put it
into the oven as well when you melt the mozzarella. I like the
pulled chicken when it isn't too warm in combination with the
hot and melted cheese.

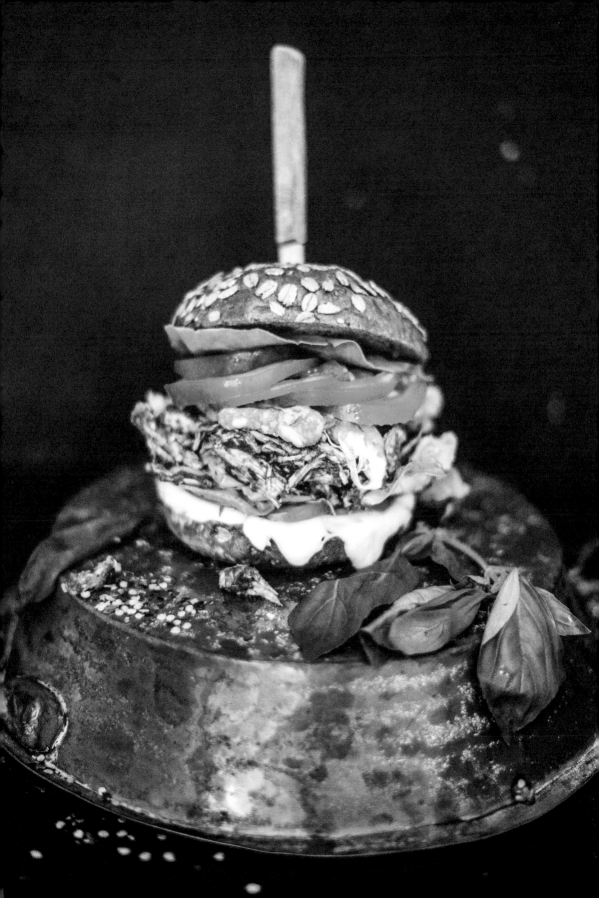

Mango & Salmon Tacos

The avocado cream that comes with these tacos is life-changing.
Have you ever had fish tacos before? If your answer is no, you'd better make
these right away.

SERVES 2 / GF, DF, RSF

TACOS
1 teaspoon dried active yeast
250–300 ml (8½–10 fl oz) lukewarm water
100 g (3½ oz) chickpea (gram) flour
100 g (3½ oz) quinoa flour or
    amaranth flour or *wholemeal spelt flour
    (*not gluten free), plus extra as required
1 teaspoon salt
coconut oil, for frying

SALMON & MARINADE
2 × approx. 200 g (7 oz) salmon fillets
2 bunches each dill and coriander
zest and juice of 1 lemon
½ teaspoon onion powder
salt and freshly ground black pepper
1–2 teaspoons maple syrup

FILLING
1 ripe mango
1 red (bell) pepper
1 red onion
2 garlic cloves
1 tablespoon olive oil
salt and freshly ground black pepper

AVOCADO CREAM
1 ripe avocado
bunch of coriander (cilantro)
1 teaspoon onion powder
1 teaspoon maple syrup
½ teaspoon chilli powder
2 tablespoons soy yoghurt
salt and freshly ground black pepper

1   For the taco shells, mix the dried yeast with the water and let it stand for about 7–8 minutes. Sift both flours and the salt into a large bowl and slowly stir in the yeast water. Transfer the mixture onto the work surface and knead into a dough with your hands. Add a little more flour if the dough is too moist and more water if the mixture is too dry.

2   Divide the dough into 6–8 equally sized portions and shape them into balls. Dust the work surface with flour. Place each ball one at a time onto the work surface, cover with parchment paper and roll out into 2–3 mm thick circles. Set the tacos aside with a piece of parchment paper between each one.

3   Preheat the oven to 160°C (320°F/Gas 3) and put a baking dish filled with water at the bottom of the oven.

4   Line a baking tray with parchment paper and add the salmon fillets on top. Mix together the ingredients for the marinade and spread over the salmon fillets.

5   For the filling, dice the mango, pepper, red onion and garlic, and mix everything together in a bowl. Drizzle the olive oil on top and season with salt and pepper. Scatter the fruit and vegetables around the salmon fillets, fold in the sides of the parchment paper and bake for 20–30 minutes.

6   In a frying pan (skillet), heat up some coconut oil on medium heat and fry the tacos on both sides until golden brown. Leave to cool over a small bowl or glass so that they get the shape of tacos.

7   For the avocado cream, put the avocado flesh into a food processor. Add the remaining ingredients and blend until smooth and creamy.

8   Take the salmon and filling out of the oven, tear the fillets into smaller pieces and divide equally with the filling into the tacos. Drizzle some of the avocado cream over each taco and serve.

VARIATION   If you don't have time to make the taco shells yourself, replace with small organic corn tacos.

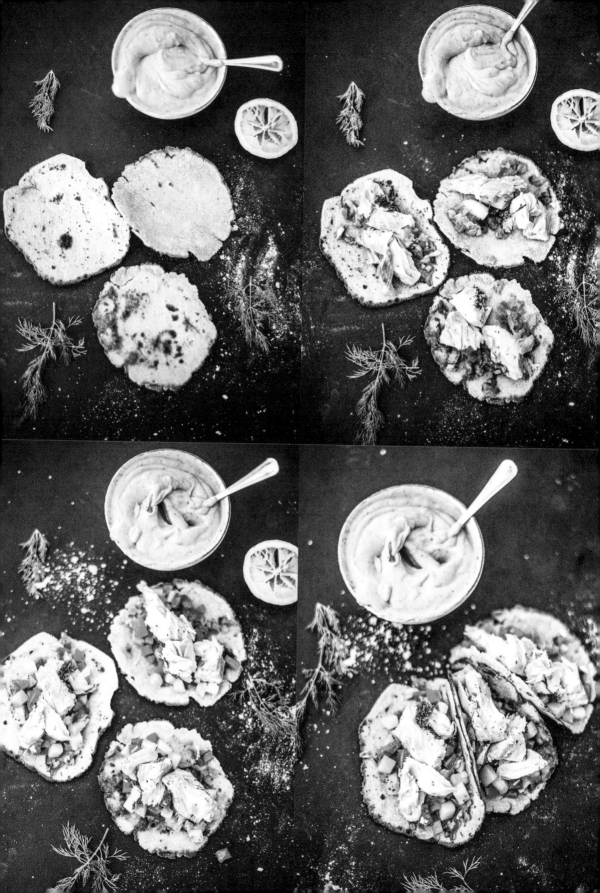

Sesame-Crusted Tuna with Broccoli Lime Cream

Every bite tastes different.

This dish is excellent to serve as a light starter and invites your guests to a completely new world of flavours. Biting into the tuna steak, you first taste the sesame crust, followed by the tuna that almost melts in your mouth. A little later the flavour of the broccoli lime cream tickles your taste buds, together with the crispy beetroot and avocado, which compliments the flavours.

SERVES 2-3 AS A STARTER / GF, DF*, RSF

TUNA STEAK

300 g (10½ oz) tuna steak

1 tablespoon olive oil

2 teaspoons lime juice

2 teaspoons maple syrup or sweetener of choice

salt and freshly ground black pepper

1 teaspoon onion powder

1 teaspoon garlic powder

4 tablespoons black sesame seeds

2 teaspoons coconut oil

BROCCOLI LIME CREAM

1 teaspoon vegetable stock (broth) powder

1 small onion, diced

200 g (7 oz) broccoli

2 tablespoons lime juice

1–2 garlic cloves

2 teaspoons maple syrup or sweetener of choice

1 tablespoon tahini

150–180 g (5–6 oz) *soy yoghurt or yoghurt of choice

salt and freshly ground black pepper

TO SERVE

1 small ripe avocado

1 small beetroot (beet)

handful of leafy salad

1   Rub the tuna steak with the olive oil, lime juice and maple syrup. Season with salt, pepper, onion powder and garlic powder.

2   For the broccoli lime cream, bring a saucepan of water to the boil, add the vegetable broth and cook the onion and broccoli for about 10 minutes until soft. Drain, then rinse with cold water and blend to a purée. Add the remaining ingredients and blend until smooth and creamy.

3   For the salad, peel the beetroot and cut into very thin slices. Boil in some water for only a few minutes so that the beetroot keeps its crunch. Drain and rinse with cold water.

4   Put the sesame seeds onto a plate and turn the tuna steak in the sesame seeds until covered completely. Heat up the coconut oil in a frying pan over a high heat, add the tuna steak and fry on both sides for 3 minutes. Take off the heat and cut into about 7 mm (½ in) thick slices. Keep the sesame seeds in the pan for later.

5   Cut the avocado in half, peel, remove the stone and cut into thin slices.

6   Put a handful of leafy salad onto a plate and top with the tuna, beetroot and avocado slices. Drizzle over the broccoli lime cream. Garnish with the fried sesame seeds left in the pan and season with some black pepper.

NOTE   This recipe is not intended to be served as a salad. The lettuce brings in some freshness, colour and is a nice garnish. If you don't want to serve any lettuce with it at all, leave it out and/or add more beetroot and avocado.

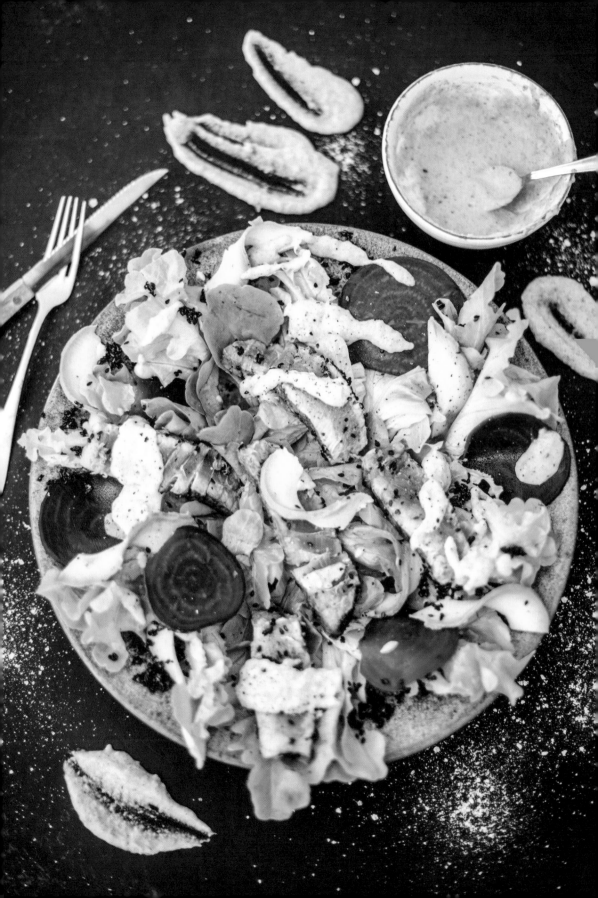

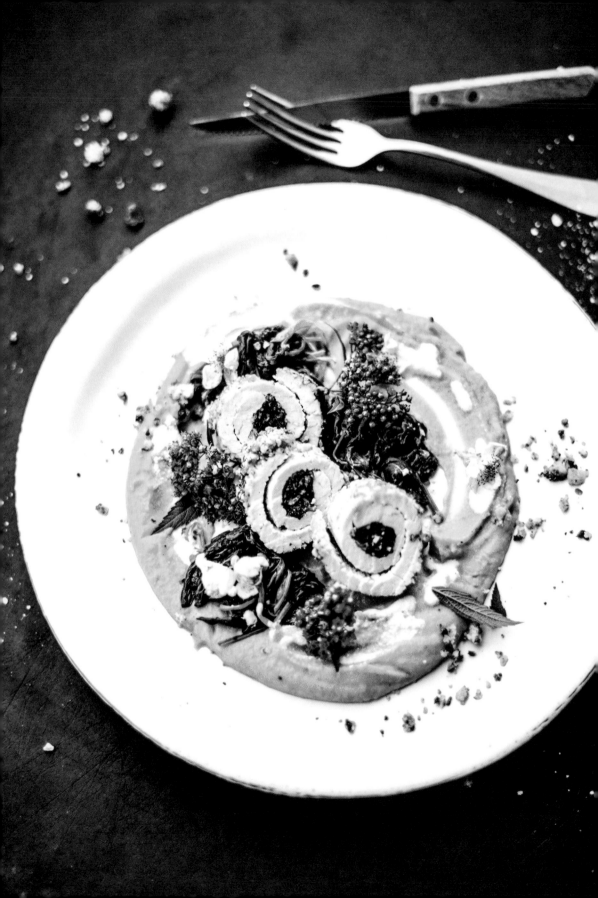

Light Sweet Potato Purée & Almond-Crusted Turkey Roulades

The purée so fluffy and light; the roulades so crunchy and delicious.
It was 9 p.m. on a Sunday night when I came up with this recipe – I was ravenous after a
late-night workout session and didn't have much left in my fridge. To add some crunch I
added an almond crust to the roulade, which makes this dish extra special.

SERVES 1-2 / GF, RSF

TURKEY ROULADES

2 turkey breasts, flattened

2 teaspoons goat's cheese

200 g (7 oz) spinach

salt and freshly ground black pepper

1 egg white

1 teaspoon almond butter

1 teaspoon maple syrup or sweetener of
choice

1 teaspoon onion powder

50–70 g (2–2½ oz) ground almonds

SWEET POTATO PURÉE

200 g (7 oz) sweet potato

1 teaspoon vegetable stock (broth) powder

1 tablespoon fresh goat's cheese

2 tablespoons soy yoghurt or yoghurt of
choice

½ teaspoon salt

½ teaspoon pepper

¼ teaspoon chilli powder

1   Preheat the oven to 180°C (350°F/Gas 4) and line a
baking tray with parchment paper.

2   Heat up some water in a saucepan, add the spinach and
cook until it has softened. Drain and press out all the excess
water. Set aside.

3   Spread the goat's cheese onto the turkey breasts, put
some of the spinach on the bottom third (reserving some)
and roll up very tight.

4   Whisk the egg white in a deep dish with the almond
butter, maple syrup and onion powder. Season with salt and
pepper and roll the turkey roulades in the mixture.

5   Add the ground almonds into another deep dish and
roll the roulades in them until covered completely. Place
on the baking tray and bake until tender in the oven for
20–30 minutes, depending on how thick your flattened
turkey breasts are. The goat's cheese will keep the meat
juicy, so it's better to leave in the oven for a few extra
minutes rather than undercook it.

6   For the sweet potato purée, bring a saucepan of
water and the vegetable stock to the boil. Peel the sweet
potatoes and chop into small pieces, then add to the vegetable
stock and cook until it is very soft and almost falling apart.
Drain and add the potato into a food processor together
with the goat's cheese and yoghurt. Add the salt, pepper
and chilli powder. Blend until smooth, creamy and light.
Return to the pan and keep warm on medium–low heat.

7   Divide the sweet potato purée neatly between plates.
Take the baked turkey roulades out of the oven and cut into
1 cm (½ in) thick slices. Lay onto the sweet potato purée,
place the remaining spinach around the roulades and serve.

VARIATION   Mix 2 teaspoons of fresh goat's cheese with
a little milk of your choice and drizzle on top.

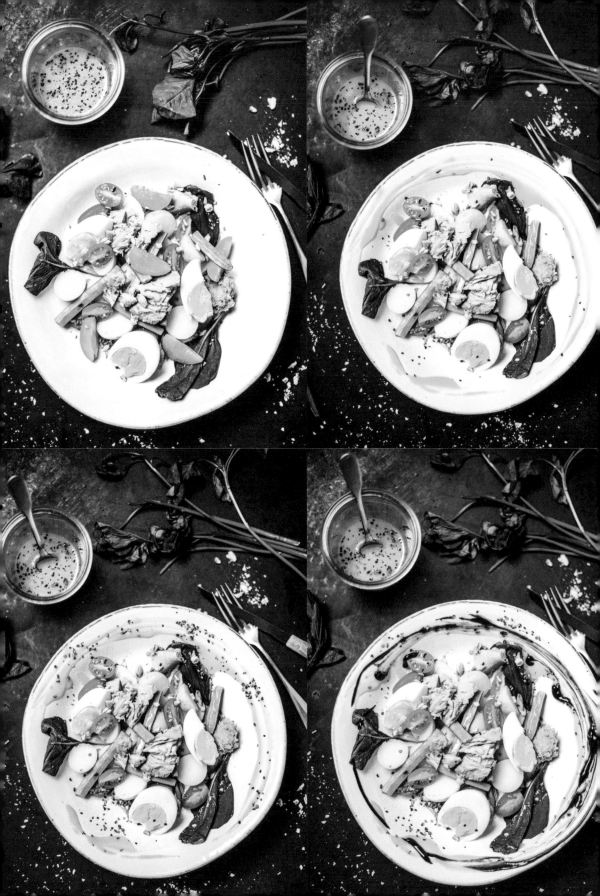

Salade Niçoise with Fresh & Fruity Mango Dressing

Almost as good as my grandma's.

The first time I ever tried salade niçoise was quite a few years ago at my grandma's. The salad blew me and my sister away! Now, whenever we visit we hope she will make this salad every time we visit. Nowhere else does it taste as good. Nevertheless, I dared to try to create my very own recipe. The ingredients are almost the same, but the dressing is completely different. Whenever you don't know if you want to eat something hot or cold, make this salad and you won't have to choose. It tastes best when eaten warm, with a cool dressing on top.

SERVES 2 / GF, DF, RSF

SALAD

2 hard-boiled eggs

8 small potatoes

2 handfuls of green beans

1 carrot

16 cherry tomatoes

1 × 160 g (5 oz) tin tuna in spring water

balsamic glaze, to serve

parsley, chives, red basil or other fresh herbs, to garnish

MANGO DRESSING

½ ripe mango

1½ tablespoons white wine vinegar

2 tablespoons olive oil

2–3 teaspoons maple syrup or sweetener of choice

½ teaspoon paprika

1 teaspoon onion powder

salt and freshly ground black pepper

1   Start by preparing the salad. Bring a saucepan of water to the boil, add the eggs and boil for 10 minutes. Remove the eggs from the pan and set aside.

2   Halve or quarter the potatoes. Cut the ends off the beans and halve. Peel the carrot and cut into batons.

3   Bring a saucepan of salted water to the boil and add the potatoes. Cook the potatoes until they are just tender, then add the beans and carrots. Cook for 3–4 minutes until the beans and carrots are still slightly crunchy. Drain and put into a bowl.

4   For the dressing, dice the mango and put it into a blender and with all the other ingredients except the salt and pepper. Blend until smooth and creamy. Pour into a bowl and season.

5   Halve the cherry tomatoes and put them into a bowl. Add the tuna and cooked vegetables and pour the dressing on top. Give it a good but careful stir.

6   Divide the salad onto plates, peel the hard-boiled eggs, cut into quarters and add on top of the salads. Drizzle over some balsamic glaze and season the salad with pepper. Garnish with herbs and sprinkle salt on top if desired.

VARIATION   Replace the potatoes with 2 medium-sized sweet potatoes. They harmonise with the mango dressing really well. Simply cut the sweet potatoes into smaller pieces and prepare just like the potatoes.

Fresh & Creamy Asparagus & Peach Salad

Light, colourful and full of flavour.

I have to admit, I wasn't always the biggest fan of asparagus, but this recipe turned me into a real asparagus lover! The way you cut vegetables and how you prepare them can make such a big difference to their taste. In this recipe I peel the asparagus and sauté the slices for a couple of minutes. The combination of sweet, bitter, crispy and creamy makes every bite a new taste experience. Ricotta, with a fat content of only around 13 percent, is a great alternative to full-fat cheese, which contains over 40 percent.

SERVES 2 / *GF, RSF

500 g (1 lb 2 oz) green asparagus

1 tablespoon olive oil

zest and juice of ½ lemon

1 teaspoon maple syrup or sweetener of choice

1 tablespoon ricotta

salt and freshly ground black pepper

1 teaspoon onion powder

½ teaspoon garlic powder

2 ripe peaches

3 tablespoons fresh ricotta cheese

2 tablespoons pine nuts

150 g (5 oz) prosciutto

drizzle of honey, to serve

2 slices of wholewheat or *gluten-free bread (optional)

1   Snap off the woody ends of the asparagus and peel into very thin slices using a vegetable peeler.

2   Heat up the olive oil in a frying pan (skillet), add the asparagus and fry for 2 minutes. Add a splash of water and steam until the water has dissolved. Take off the heat and tip into a bowl.

3   Add the lemon zest and juice, maple syrup and ricotta to the asparagus. Season with salt, pepper, onion powder and garlic powder, and stir until well combined.

4   Dice the peaches. Add to the asparagus and stir again.

5   Toast the pine nuts in a frying pan over a medium heat until golden brown. Take off the heat and leave to cool.

6   Divide the asparagus salad onto plates, tear the prosciutto slices into pieces, add on top of the salads, spoon on the remaining ricotta and sprinkle over the pine nuts.

7   Season with some black pepper, add a drizzle of honey and serve the salad lukewarm. If desired, serve with 2 slices of wholewheat bread.

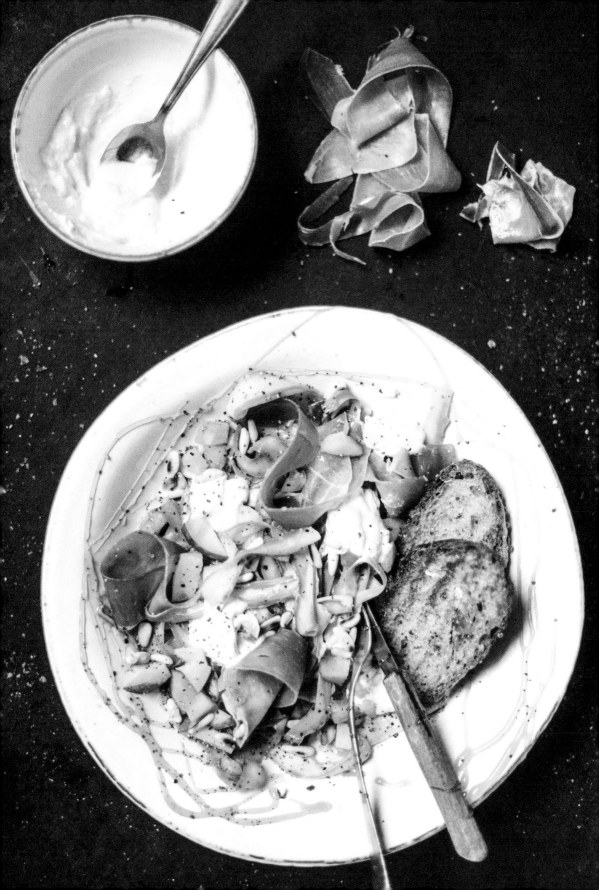

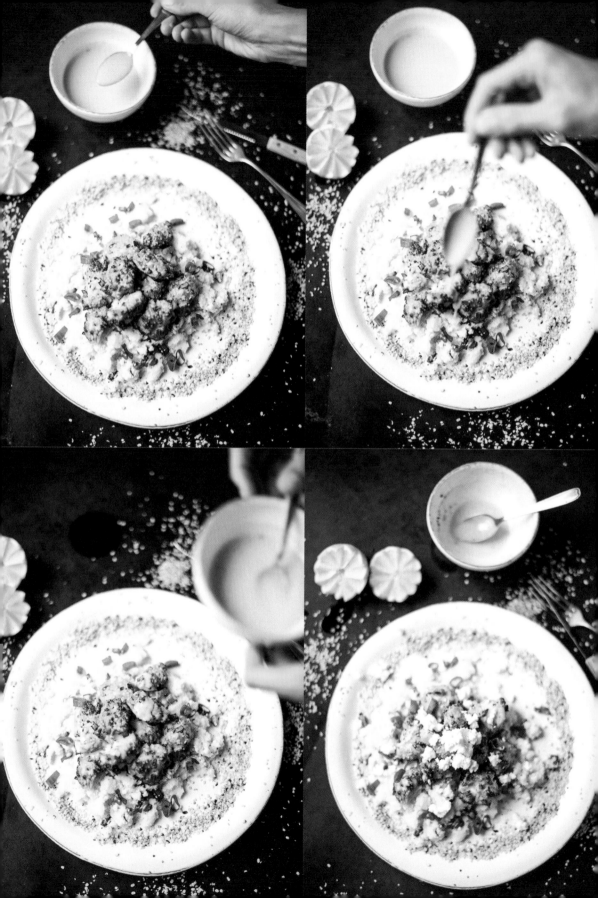

Couscous & Hemp Heart-Crusted Chicken with Lemon Honey Sauce

A dish that fills you up with all you need.
The juicy chicken in a light and nutty hemp heart crust is served with the most refreshing and slightly sweet lemon sauce and a good portion of fluffy couscous. If you want, add some crumbled feta on top – it really enhances the flavours in the dish.

SERVES 2 / DF, RSF

CHICKEN
400 g (14 oz) chicken breast
2 tablespoons cornflour (cornstarch)
1 egg white
salt and freshly ground black pepper
1–2 tablespoons honey
1 tablespoon almond butter
zest and juice of 2 lemons
½ tablespoon tamari or soy sauce
1 teaspoon onion powder
1 teaspoon garlic powder
4 tablespoons hemp hearts

COUSCOUS
120–150 g (4–5 oz) couscous
100–150 ml (3½–5 fl oz) water
1 teaspoon salt
2 spring onions (scallions), chopped
olive oil
zest and juice of 1 small lemon

LEMON SAUCE
zest and juice of 2 lemons
2 tablespoons honey
2 teaspoons almond butter
200 ml (7 fl oz) milk of choice,
    e.g. soy, almond, rice milk
salt and freshly ground black pepper
1 teaspoon onion powder
1 teaspoon garlic powder

TO SERVE
hemp hearts
1 spring onion (scallion), chopped
feta (optional)

1   Preheat the oven to 200°C (400°F/Gas 6) and line a baking tray with parchment paper.

2   Cut the chicken breasts into bite-sized pieces. Line up four deep plates. Pour the cornflour into the first plate. In the second plate, whisk together the egg white, salt and pepper. To the third plate, add the honey, almond butter, lemon zest and juice, tamari, onion powder and garlic powder. And to plate number four, add the hemp hearts.

3   Coat the chicken pieces in all of the four plates' contents sequentially. Once the chicken is covered in the hemp heart crust, place onto the baking tray and bake for 20–25 minutes until golden brown and tender.

4   For the lemon sauce, put all the ingredients into a saucepan and bring to the boil. Reduce the heat to low and cook for about 10 minutes. The sauce will thicken a bit. Stir from time to time and add a splash of milk if the mixture starts to become too thick.

5   For the couscous, bring the water to the boil with the couscous and salt and cook for 2 minutes. Turn off the heat, cover and leave it to swell for a few minutes. Loosen the couscous with a fork, add the spring onions, olive oil, lemon juice and zest, and stir until well combined.

6   Take the baked chicken pieces out of the oven. Spoon the couscous onto plates and place the chicken on top of the couscous. Drizzle over a good amount of the lemon sauce, garnish with hemp hearts, chopped spring onion and crumbled feta, if using.

Beef Tenderloin with Plum Blackberry Sauce & Garlic Mushrooms

I can never get enough of this dish!

A good piece of local organic meat has its price, but for a recipe like this it's absolutely worth it. I'd rather eat good quality meat very rarely than eat mid-grade meat daily. The fruity sauce pairs wonderfully with the beef. You might not have had a sauce like this with meat yet, but I'm sure you'll be convinced. As a light side dish, I made some garlic mushrooms with fresh spinach. I could eat this every single day, to be honest. And if garlic didn't have such a strong aftertaste, I would probably add around five more cloves of garlic right away!

— SERVES 2 / GF, DF —

BEEF TENDERLOIN

300 g (10½ oz) beef tenderloin

1 tablespoon olive oil

salt and freshly ground black pepper

GARLIC MUSHROOMS

1–2 teaspoons coconut oil

2 garlic cloves, chopped

200 g (7 oz) button mushrooms

200 g (7 oz) spinach

1 spring onion (scallion), chopped

few springs of parsley, chopped

salt and freshly ground black pepper

SAUCE

150 ml (5 fl oz) water

1 teaspoon vegetable stock (broth) powder

4–5 plums, fresh or frozen

1 small red onion

4–6 dates, pitted

150 g (5 oz) blackberries

100 ml (3½ fl oz) red wine

salt and freshly ground black pepper

1 teaspoon garlic powder

2–3 teaspoons maple syrup

1   For the sauce, bring the water and vegetable stock to the boil in a saucepan. Halve and stone the plums. Peel and halve the onion. Add the plums, onion, dates and blackberries to the pan and cook over a high heat for 3–4 minutes. Once slightly reduced, add the red wine. Cook for another few minutes, season with salt, pepper, onion powder and maple syrup and turn down the heat to low–medium. Cook for at least 15 minutes until the sauce thickens.

2   To make the garlic mushrooms, in a frying pan (skillet), heat up the coconut oil, add the garlic and fry until shiny. Add the mushrooms, spinach, spring onion and parsley. Season and cook until the water from the vegetables has evaporated. Turn off the heat and cover with a lid.

3   To cook the beef, heat up a frying pan or griddle pan. Rub the beef tenderloin with the olive oil and season with salt and pepper. Place into the pan and cook to the desired core temperature: rare 40–44°C (104–111°F); medium 48–52°C (118–126°F); well done 52–54°C (126–129°F). Take off the heat, wrap in aluminum foil to keep the beef warm and let it rest for a few minutes.

4   Cut the beef tenderloin into slices and serve together with the garlic mushrooms and spinach. Serve the sauce separately.

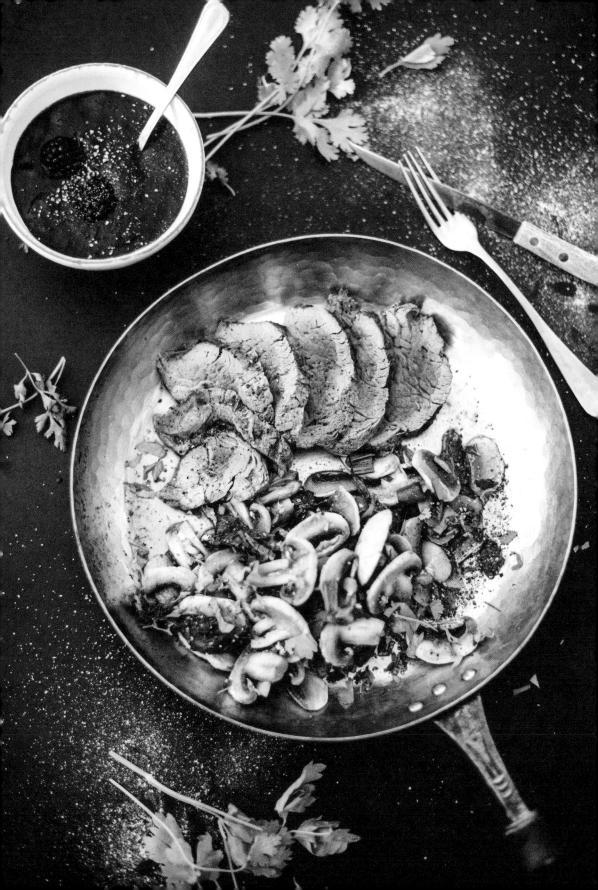

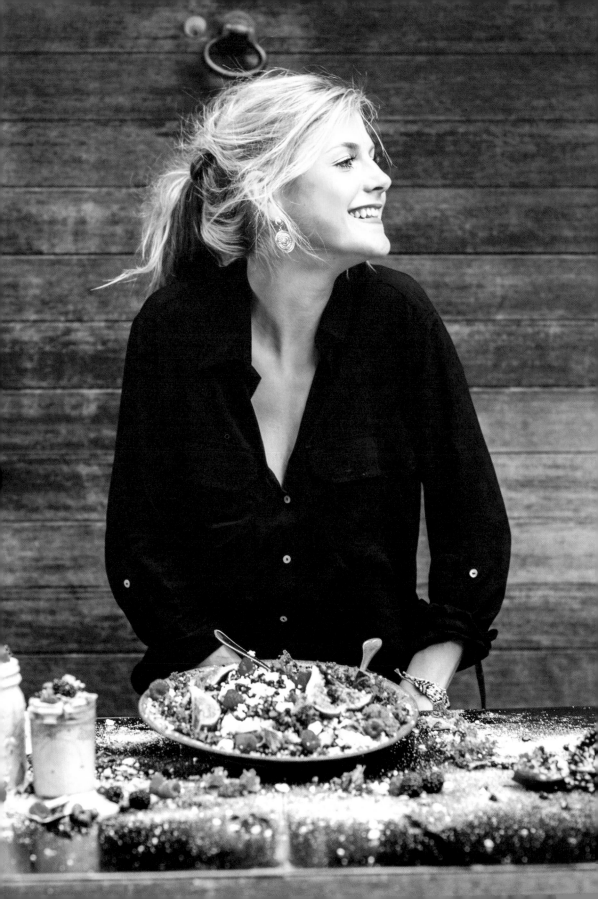

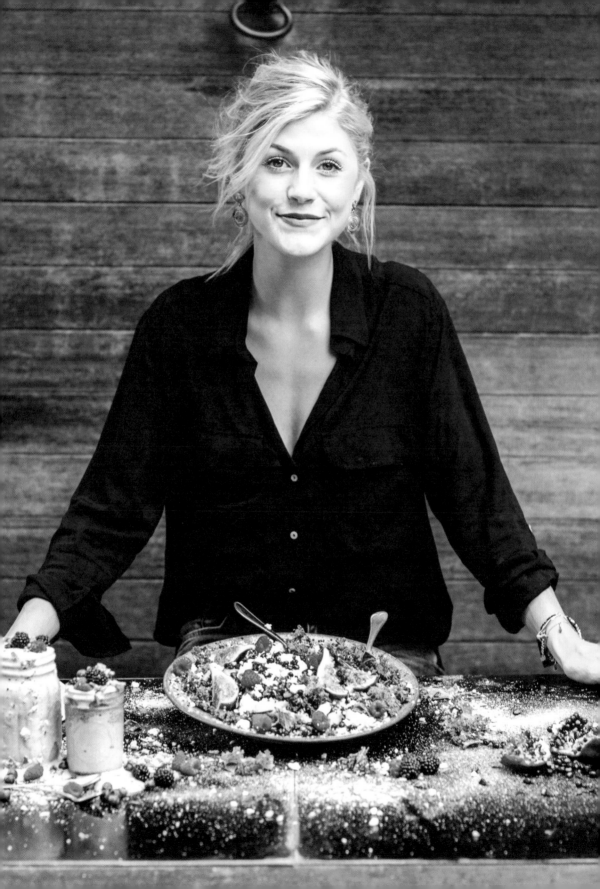

Colourful Kale Salad with Berries, Figs & Feta

A salad that makes your heart beat faster.

The taste and all the different colours in this salad will be sure to win you over. Salads can be so boring and tasteless, or they can be better than any warm dish! In this case, I enjoy every single bite, I pick every crumb out of the bowl and when it's empty, I try to get all the leftover dressing onto my fork. This salad has it all: it's creamy, crispy and crunchy, fruity, salty and juicy, and has a light, refreshing aroma. Kale contains plenty of good nutrients and is very versatile. You can add it into your smoothie, have it as a salad like in this recipe or even make kale chips (see page 197). The kale itself is quite tough and stringy, so it's really important to massage the dressing into the leaves for a few minutes so that they wilt and take on the flavour of the dressing.

SERVES 2-3 / GF, DF*, V, VGN*, RSF

KALE SALAD

400 g (14 oz) kale

150 g (5 oz) feta

1 ripe avocado

seeds of ½ pomegranate

4 figs, quartered

250 g (9 oz) fresh or frozen and thawed raspberries

2 tablespoons almonds

1 tablespoon pecans, crushed

honey, to serve

lemon juice, to serve

DRESSING

2 tablespoons olive oil

2 tablespoons white wine vinegar

zest and juice of 1 lemon

1 teaspoon onion powder

1 teaspoon garlic powder

1 tablespoon peanut or almond butter

2–3 teaspoons maple syrup or sweetener of choice

salt and freshly ground black pepper

1 Remove the tough stems from the kale leaves. Tear the leaves into bite-sized pieces, then wash, drain and tip into a large bowl.

2 Add all the ingredients for the dressing into a separate bowl and whisk until well combined. Drizzle over the kale leaves and massage the leaves with your hands for 2–3 minutes until they are shiny and have wilted. Try a bite and if the leaves are still too tough, massage them for a little longer.

3 Crumble the feta over the kale. Halve and peel the avocado, remove the stone, dice and add it to the salad as well as the pomegranate seeds. Stir until well combined.

4 Toast the nuts in a dry frying pan (skillet) over a medium heat until golden brown. Take off the heat and let them cool, then crush them in a mortar.

5 Divide the salad between plates and top with the figs, raspberries, crushed almonds and pecans. Drizzle over some lemon juice and honey for some extra freshness and sweetness. And now, enjoy every single bite. Don't forget to pick out all the crumbs left in the bowl!

VARIATIONS   *For the dairy-free and vegan option, don't add feta – replace with grilled tofu, and use maple syrup instad of honey. For a reduced-fat version, add ricotta or cottage cheese instead of feta.

FROZEN RASPBERRIES   If you use frozen raspberries, thaw them completely in cold water, drain, then add.

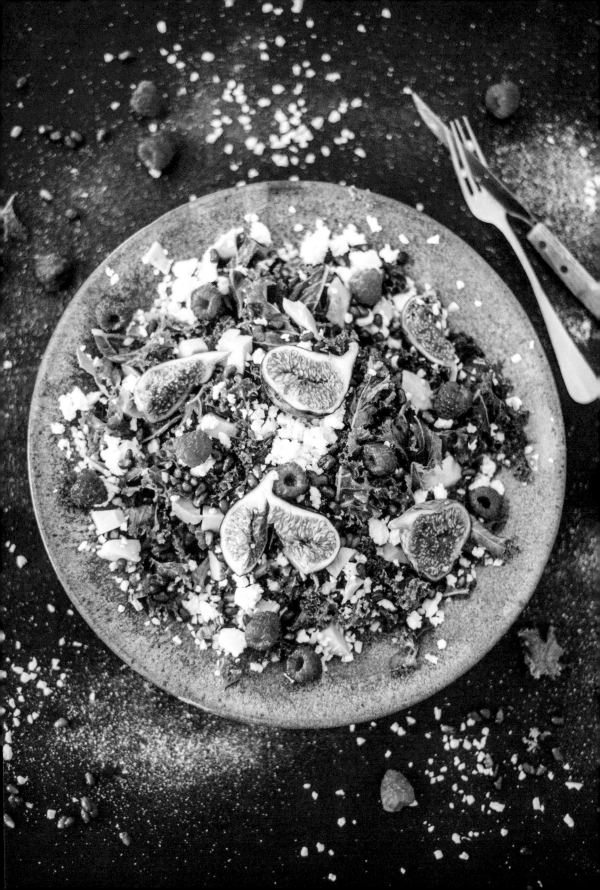

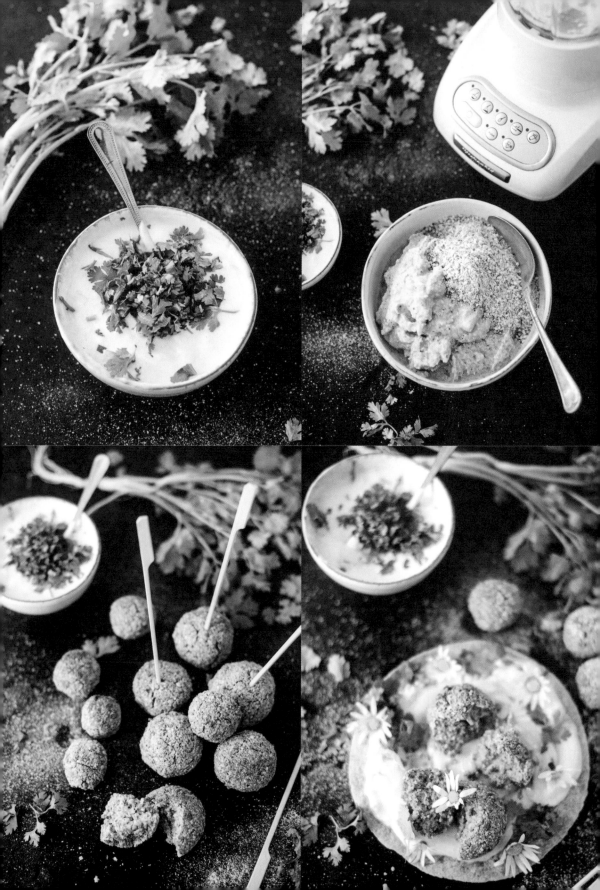

Almond-Crusted Pea & Edamame Balls with Tzatziki

Love at first taste.

These baked pea balls have a light and crunchy almond crust and are fluffy, light and simply irresistible! Together with the tzatziki, which I usually make with low-fat Greek yoghurt and fat-reduced natural yoghurt, this dish is perfect to serve as an appetiser. If you want to have it as a meal, spread some tzatziki on a wholewheat tortilla, add some of the pea-edamame balls, your favourite salad, and wrap up!

—————————————— MAKES 10-14 BALLS / GF, V, RSF ——————————————

PEA & EDAMAME BALLS

120 g (4 oz) frozen peas

4 tablespoons fresh or frozen and thawed edamame

1 garlic clove

1 teaspoon onion powder

salt and freshly ground black pepper

1 teaspoon maple syrup or sweetener of choice

1 egg

dash of milk of choice, e.g. soy, almond, rice milk (optional)

3 tablespoons ground almonds

COATING

1 egg

1 egg white

4 tablespoons ground almonds

1 teaspoon onion powder

salt and freshly ground black pepper

TZATZIKI

1 small cucumber

150 g (5 oz) low-fat Greek yoghurt

150 g (5 oz) natural yoghurt

bunch of coriander (cilantro), chopped

zest and juice of ½ lemon

salt and freshly ground black pepper

1 teaspoon onion powder

1 teaspoon garlic powder

1   Preheat the oven to 180°C (350°F/Gas 4). Line a baking tray with parchment paper. Take the frozen peas and edamame out of the freezer and allow to thaw.

2   For the tzatziki, peel and grate the cucumber. Squeeze out the excess water with your hands. Add to a bowl with all the remaining ingredients, stir well and cool in the fridge.

3   To make the pea balls, put all the ingredients except the almonds into a food processor and blend to a thick mixture. Add a dash of your choice of milk if the mixture is too thick.

4   Spoon the pea mixture into a bowl, add the ground almonds and stir until well combined. With your hands, form 10–14 equally sized balls.

5   Prepare the coating by whisking the egg with the egg white in a deep plate. In another deep plate, mix the ground almonds, onion powder, salt and pepper.

6   Coat the balls in the egg mixture first, then in the almond mixture until completely covered. Lay them onto the prepared baking tray.

7   Bake in the middle of the oven for 20–30 minutes until the crust is golden brown. Take out of the oven, let them cool for a few minutes and serve with the cooled tzatziki.

TIP   You can double the quantities and freeze half of the prepared balls. Then you'll have a delicious appetiser ready for your guests in moments by simply baking the frozen balls at 180°C (350°F/Gas 4) for 20 minutes. While they're baking, you have enough time to make a tzatziki to serve with it.

Roasted Sweet Potato Tartlet with Sage & Date Hummus

A recipe that nobody can resist making.

I'm sure most of you have had hummus before. Many times, probably. But have you ever had date hummus? I fell in love with it right from the start and could barely keep my hands off it! The combination of sweet and savoury gives this dish the perfect kick. A must-try for all hummus lovers. It goes so well with this simple yet delicious tartlet. Definitely a recipe for the autumn.

SERVES 2 (1 TARTLET – APPROX. 20 CM/8 IN) / GF, DF, V, VGN, RSF

TARTLET

3 medium-sized sweet potatoes

2 apples

2 red onions

1 tablespoon coconut oil, melted, or olive oil

salt and freshly ground black pepper

1 teaspoon onion powder

handful of sage leaves

DATE HUMMUS

5–6 Medjool dates

250 g (9 oz) chickpeas (garbanzos), cooked or soaked

1 tablespoon tahini

1 tablespoon peanut or almond butter

1 garlic clove or 2 teaspoons garlic powder

1 tablespoon olive oil

1½ tablespoons lemon juice

100 ml (3½ fl oz) milk of choice, e.g. soy, almond, rice milk

salt and freshly ground black pepper

1   Preheat the oven to 180°C (350°F/Gas 4) and line a round baking tray with baking parchment.

2   For the tartlet, wash the sweet potatoes and cut off the ends. Wash the apples and peel the onion. Cut everything into 1–2 mm thick slices and layer on the baking tray in a circle, working from the outside to the inside. Drizzle the melted coconut oil or olive oil on top, and season with salt, pepper and onion powder. Tear the sage leaves into small pieces and sprinkle on top of the tartlet.

3   Bake for 25–35 minutes until the edges of the sweet potato, apple and onion slices have browned and become slightly crisp.

4   For the hummus, put the dates into a bowl, pour boiling water on top and let them stand for about 10 minutes. Place the remaining ingredients, except the salt and pepper, into a food processor and blend to a smooth consistency. Drain the dates, add to the hummus and blend again for a minute or two until creamy. Season with salt and pepper.

5   Take the tartlet out of the oven and serve with the date hummus. I always like to add a drizzle of honey and lemon juice on top, but it's totally up to you whether you want to do the same or not!

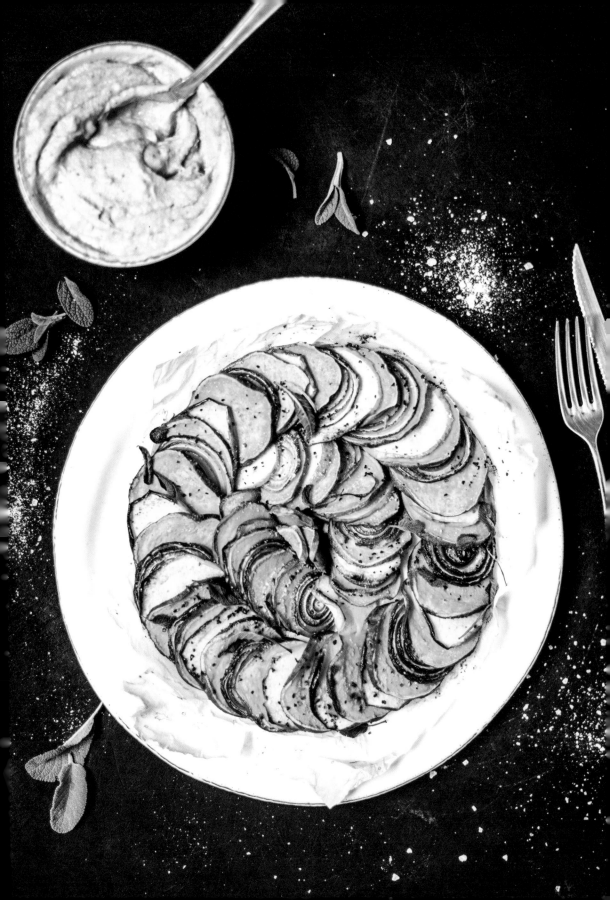

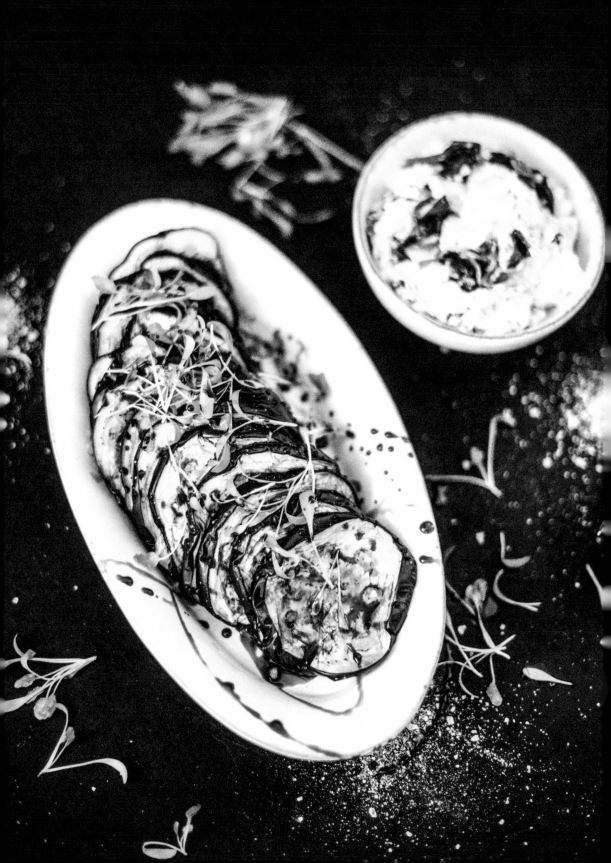

Roasted Aubergine with Spinach & Artichoke Dip

I officially declare aubergine as my favourite vegetable.
Aubergine (eggplant) all day, every day – I wouldn't mind it. Only if it's well prepared though! I prefer them either roasted or grilled, and it's important to drizzle some good-quality olive oil on top before doing this. The oil gives the aubergine that juicy, soft flesh that almost melts in your mouth and tastes delicious. The balsamic glaze drizzled on top gives it an Italian touch and adds sweetness. And this dip... I won't even start. Simply try it – it's honestly incredible!

SERVES 2 OR 4 AS A STARTER / GF, V, RSF

ROASTED AUBERGINE

2 large aubergines (eggplants)

2 teaspoons onion powder

1 teaspoon garlic powder

salt and freshly ground black pepper

1–2 tablespoons olive oil

balsamic glaze, to serve

cress, to garnish

SPINACH & ARTICHOKE DIP

3–4 tablespoons water

1 teaspoon vegetable stock (broth) powder

150 g (5 oz) spinach

6 artichoke hearts in salted water, drained

2 teaspoons onion powder

1–2 teaspoons garlic powder

250 g (9 oz) ricotta

lemon juice

salt and freshly ground black pepper

1   Preheat the oven to 180°C (350°F/Gas 4). Line 2 baking trays with parchment paper.

2   Cut the ends off the aubergines, and cut into 1–1.5 cm (½–¾ in) thick slices. Lay the slices out on the baking trays, season with onion powder, garlic powder, salt and pepper, drizzle the olive oil on top and roast in the middle of the oven for 20–25 minutes until golden brown and soft.

3   While the aubergines are roasting in the oven, prepare the dip. In a smal saucepan, bring the water and vegetable stock to a boil, add the spinach, lower the heat and cook for a few minutes until wilted. Take off the heat, drain well and put the spinach into a bowl. Chop the artichoke hearts into small pieces and add them to the spinach with the onion powder, garlic powder, ricotta and lemon juice. Stir until well combined and season with salt and pepper. Taste and add another drizzle of lemon juice if desired.

4   Take the aubergines out of the oven, arrange them beautifully onto plates, drizzle the balsamic glaze on top, garnish with some fresh cress and serve with the dip.

TIP   Serve this dish as a starter for four people. The dip also tastes great with other roasted vegetables like courgette or pumpkin.

Refreshing Bulgur Salad with Tomato, Avocado & Cranberries

A Middle Eastern salad that will make your belly jump for joy.
A refreshing cleanser for the palate, that's what you get from this salad.
You and your guests are going to love it. It can be enjoyed during any season and will always be a hit because it's fresh, fruity and filling. Bulgur is a wholewheat grain made out of durum wheat. In the Middle East, bulgur has the same status that pasta has in Italy. It's used for many traditional dishes such as tabbouleh.

SERVES 2-3 / DF, V, VGN, RSF

BULGUR SALAD
225–280 ml (8–9¾ fl oz) water
1 teaspoon vegetable stock (broth) powder
8–10 tablespoons bulgur
1 ripe avocado
1 spring onion (scallion)
2 bunches of parsley, plus extra to serve
300 g (10½ oz) cherry tomatoes
2 tablespoons unsweetened cranberries
3 tablespoons roasted and crushed almonds

DRESSING
1 tablespoon olive oil
1 tablespoon almond butter
1–2 tablespoons white balsamic vinegar
2 tablespoons lemon juice
2 teaspoons maple syrup or sweetener of choice
1 teaspoon onion powder
1 teaspoon garlic powder
½ teaspoon chilli powder
salt and freshly ground black pepper

1   Bring the water, vegetable broth and bulgur to the boil. Cook for 2 minutes and reduce the heat to medium–low. Simmer for about 10 minutes, take off the heat, put into a bowl and leave to cool.

2   Cut the avocado in half, remove the stone, peel, dice and add to the cooked bulgur. Finely chop the spring onion and parsley and cut the tomatoes into quarters. Toast the almonds in a dry frying pan (skillet) over a medium heat until golden brown. Take off the heat, let them cool and then crush them. Keep 1 tablespoon of the almonds for later. Add all the remaining salad ingredients to the bulgur and stir well.

3   For the dressing, add all the ingredients, except the salt and pepper, into a bowl and whisk until well combined. Season to taste.

4   Drizzle the dressing on top of the bulgur salad and stir for a couple of minutes until well combined.

5   Spoon onto plates, garnish with fresh parsley and sprinkle the reserved crushed almonds on top. Serve immediately or cool in the fridge for 1–2 hours.

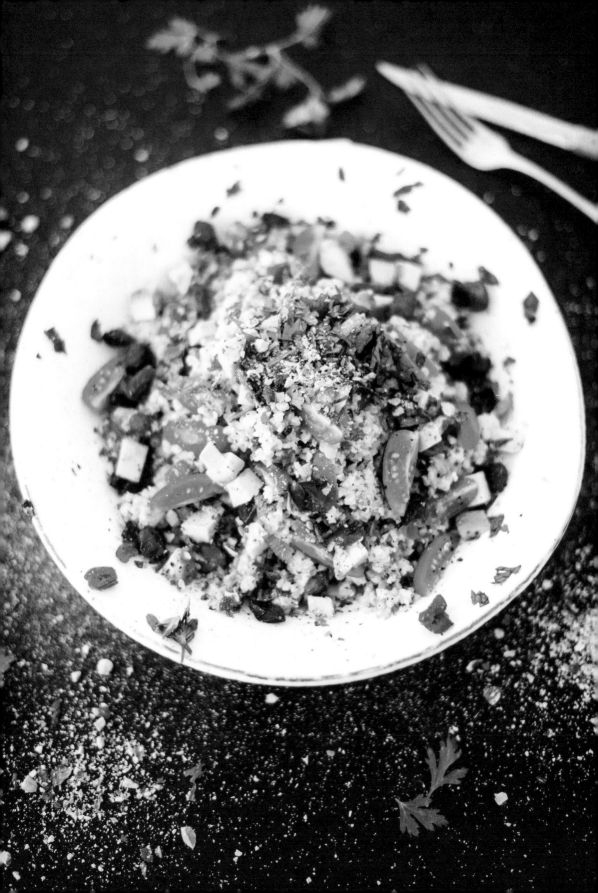

Spring Rolls with Spicy Mango, Chilli & Peanut Sauce

The healthy version of fast finger food.

The first time I made these spring rolls wasn't that long ago, but ever since then I eat them at least once a week. I also love to make them when I have friends over. They are easy to share – everybody can have as much as they want because you can make more in no time. The avocado in the filling and peanut butter in the sauce (I could eat this dressing with a spoon just like a soup. Yes, it's that good!) provide healthy fats that our body needs to function properly. Bon appetit!

SERVES 2-4 / GF, DF, V, VGN, RSF

10–12 large rice paper sheets

FILLING

1 ripe avocado

1 cucumber

2 carrots

1 ripe mango

1 small red cabbage

1 small iceberg or round lettuce

bunch of Thai basil

MANGO CHILLI PEANUT SAUCE

1 ripe mango

100 ml (3½ fl oz) milk of choice, e.g. soy, almond, rice milk

100 ml (3½ fl oz) coconut milk

1–3 teaspoons chilli powder (depending on how spicy you like it)

½ teaspoon curry powder

1 small onion

1 teaspoon garlic powder

1 tablespoon lime juice

2 teaspoons maple syrup or sweetener of choice

2 tablespoons peanut butter

salt and freshly ground black pepper

1 Cut the avocado in half, remove the stone, peel, dice and drizzle some lime juice on top. Peel the cucumber and carrot, then cut into very thin batons or peel with a julienne peeler. Peel the mango, cut the flesh off the pit and cut into thin slices. Finely slice the red cabbage. Wash and drain the lettuce and tear into smaller pieces.

2 Add some lukewarm water into a large saucepan and soak one rice paper sheet in it for about 10 seconds. Transfer onto the work surface. (Make one roll at a time and don't soak all the rice paper sheets at once, otherwise they will become too soft.)

3 Spread some of the vegetables across the lower two thirds of the rice paper sheet. Leave some space around the edges. Add some salad leaves first, then a few cucumber and carrot sticks, a little bit of red cabbage, about two mango and avocado pieces each and finish off with some Thai basil leaves. First, fold in the bottom of the rice paper, then tuck in the sides and roll up tight. Repeat with the other rice paper sheets until you have used up all of the filling.

4 For the mango sauce, peel the mango and cut off the flesh. Put into a food processor with the remaining ingredients and blend to a smooth, creamy and slightly thick paste. Taste and add extra chilli powder if you want the sauce to be spicier. Garnish with more chilli.

5 Cut the salad rolls in half and fold a salad leaf around the rolls to prevent them from sticking together. It is the easiest way to eat the rolls and additional greens are never a bad thing! Serve with the dipping sauce and enjoy.

TIP Be careful rolling up the rice paper rolls and don't add too much filling – the sheets can tear very easily.

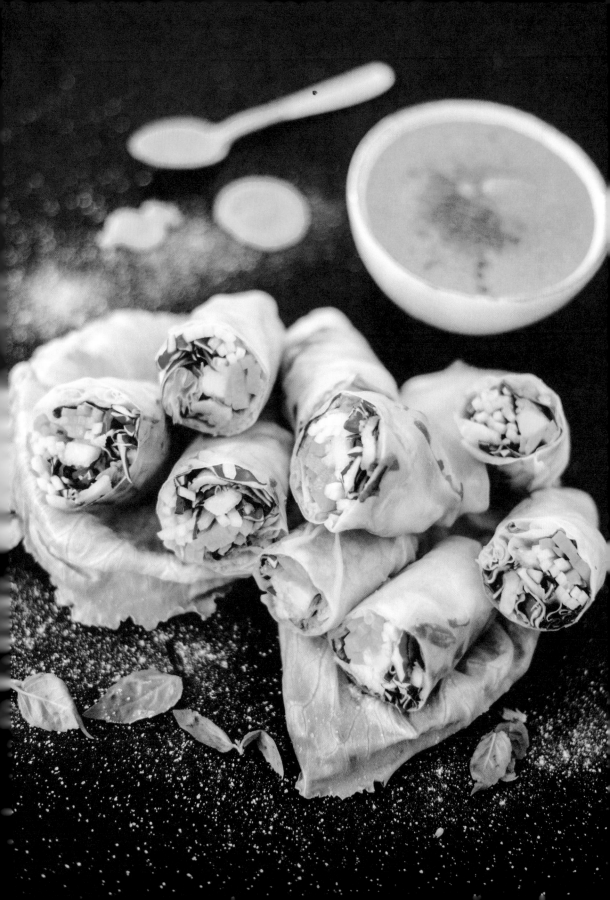

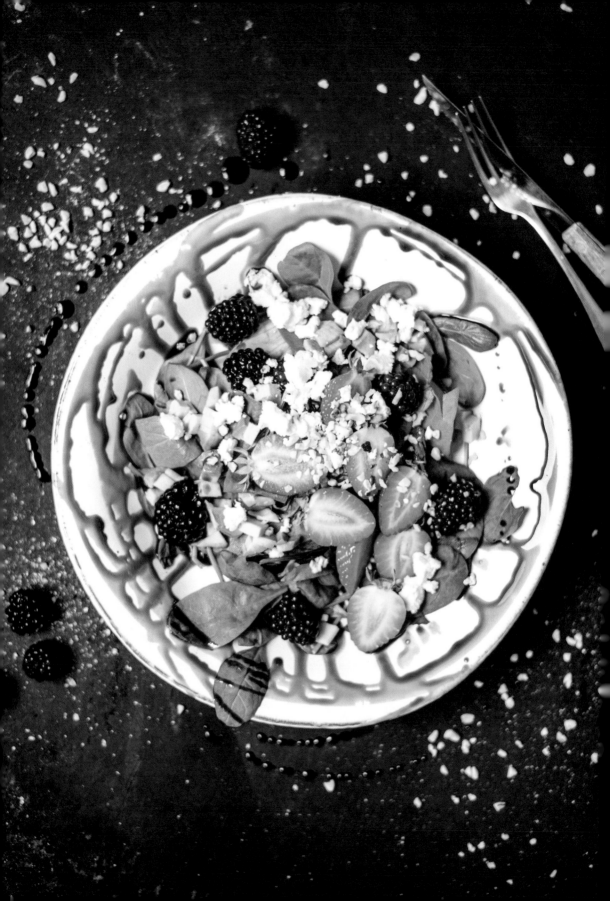

Simple Spinach Salad with Berries, Feta & Avocado

... and an extremely tasty hazelnut balsamic dressing.

I love making salads because you can get so creative with the ingredients, so they never taste exactly the same. This hazelnut balsamic dressing is absolutely mindblowing! Adding berries to a salad not only provides colour, but also a fresh, fruity and sweet taste. This dish makes a light but filling lunch or dinner. Oh, and don't forget to roast the hazelnuts – it makes such a difference.

SERVES 2 / GF, V, RSF

SALAD

500 g (1 lb 2 oz) fresh spinach

1 ripe avocado

200 g (7 oz) fresh or frozen and thawed blackberries

100 g (3½ oz) feta

DRESSING

40–60 g (1½–2 oz) hazelnuts

1 tablespoon olive oil

2 tablespoons balsamic vinegar

1–2 teaspoons maple syrup or sweetener

salt and freshly ground black pepper

dash of almond or soy milk

large handful of fresh strawberries, to serve

balsamic glaze, to serve

1   Roast the hazelnuts in the oven at 160°C (320°F/Gas 3) for about 15 minutes. Take out of the oven and let them cool.

2   Wash the spinach and dry it off with kitchen towel or using a salad spinner. Put it into a large bowl. Cut the avocado in half, remove the stone, peel and dice, and add to the spinach. Crumble in the feta and add the blackberries.

3   For the dressing, put 30–40 g (1–1½ oz) of the hazelnuts along with the remaining ingredients into a blender and blend until smooth and creamy. This might take a few minutes. If the mixture is too thick, simply add a dash of milk and blend again.

4   Pour the dressing over of the salad and stir until well combined so that every salad leaf is shiny. Serve onto plates.

5   Garnish with fresh strawberries, then crush the remaining hazelnuts and sprinkle on top of the salad. Finish off with a drizzle of balsamic glaze.

VARIATION   If you don't have time to roast the hazelnuts in the oven, toast them in a frying pan (skillet) over a medium heat until golden brown. Take off the heat and let them cool for a bit, then crush.

Cauliflower Rice with Sweet Thai Sauce

When cauliflower turns into rice.

Last year, when I was travelling around Thailand for a month, I ate the typical fried rice dish quite a lot. The taste was always a winner, but to me there weren't enough vegetables for such a big portion of rice. Back in Switzerland I wanted to make a similar dish in terms of taste, but add more vegetables. The idea of replacing the rice with grated cauliflower didn't leave my mind, so I tried it. In combination with this sauce it's just amazing. You can really stuff yourself with this dish because it's mainly composed of vegetables.

SERVES 3 / DF, RSF

1 large cauliflower

salt and freshly ground black pepper

3 medium carrots

1 medium sweet potato
  or 200 g (7 oz) pumpkin

2 teaspoons coconut oil

120 g (4 oz) peas

120 g (4 oz) sweetcorn

1 egg

2 egg whites

1 tablespoon tamari or soy sauce, plus extra
  to serve

2 teaspoons fish sauce

2 teaspoons oyster sauce

1 tablespoon maple syrup or sweetener
  of choice

1 teaspoon curry powder

1 teaspoon mild or spicy paprika

salt and freshly ground black pepper

6–8 kaffir lime leaves (available at every
  Asian store; otherwise add some lime peel
  and juice instead)

chilli powder (optional)

1   Cut the stalk off the cauliflower, tear it into smaller pieces and grate by hand or with a food processor. Season with salt, stir and set aside. Peel and dice the carrots and sweet potato.

2   Heat up the coconut oil in a large frying pan (skillet) or wok, add the carrot and sweet potato and fry for about 5–7 minutes. Stir in the grated cauliflower, peas and sweetcorn and fry for another 5–7 minutes.

3   In a small bowl, whisk the egg, egg white and 1 tablespoon of tamari. Add to the vegetables, stir well and lower the heat. Stir in the remaining ingredients one by one. Before adding the kaffir lime leaves, remove the stems, finely crumble the leaves and then add. Turn up the heat again and fry for 2–3 minutes, add some more tamari or chilli if you like it spicy, stir well, take off the heat and serve into bowls.

TIP   This 'rice' dish can easily be stored in an airtight container for up to 3 days without losing its taste. You can either enjoy it cold as a salad or heat it up again. If you heat it up again you might have to add a bit more moisture by adding another splash of tamari, fish sauce or oyster sauce and a drizzle of honey.

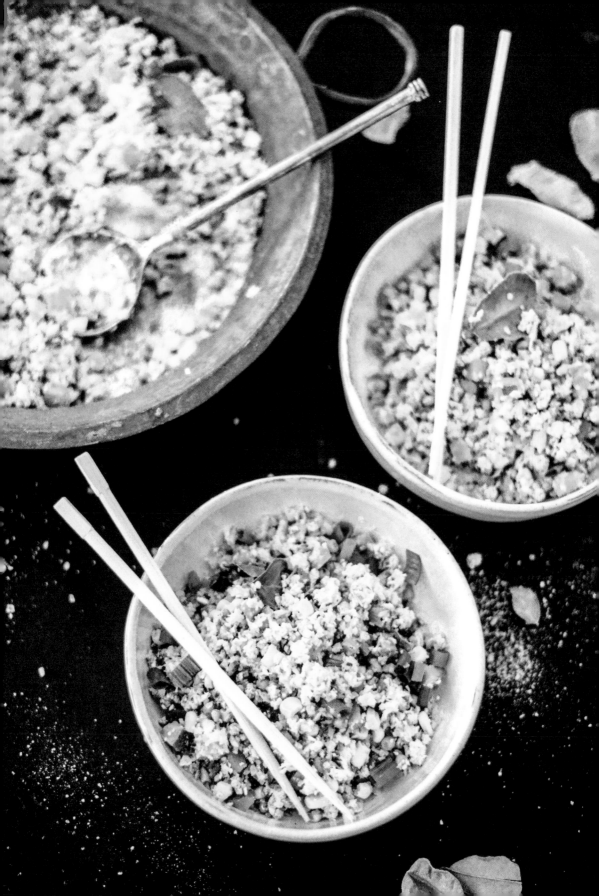

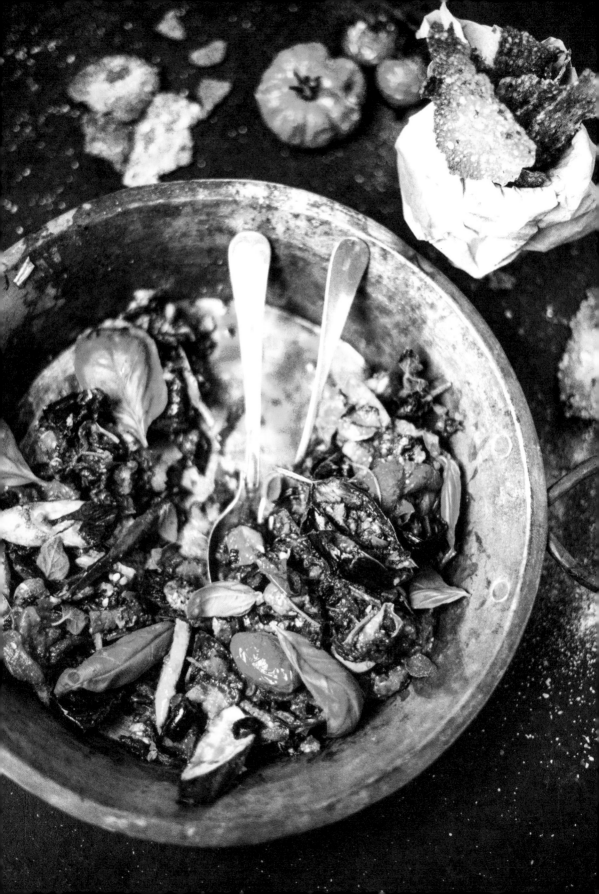

Caponata alla Nadia with Oregano Corn Crackers

... a lot of amore and a pinch of Italia.

In this dish, the veggies show off their real talent and prove what they're capable of. Even though the caponata tastes great on its own, I wanted to make something to accompany it, to add some crunch and good carbohydrates. These thin and crispy corn crackers seemed just perfect.

SERVES 2–3 / GF, V, RSF

CAPONATA

2 aubergines (eggplants)

3 courgettes (zucchinis)

500 g (1 lb 2 oz) tomatoes

500 g (1 lb 2 oz) button mushrooms

2–3 tablespoons olive oil

salt and freshly ground black pepper

2 teaspoons onion powder

1 spring onion (scallion), chopped

2 garlic cloves, chopped

½ red chilli

2–3 bunches of fresh oregano, leaves

3–4 handful spinach, fresh

4 tablespoons tomato purée (paste)

1–2 tablespoons balsamic glaze

3 tablespoons black olives, pitted

2 teaspoons maple syrup or sweetener

20–40 g (¾–1½ oz) Parmesan, grated

basil, to garnish

CORN CRACKERS

400 ml (13 fl oz) water

2–3 teaspoons vegetable stock (broth) powder

100 g (3½ oz) cornmeal

small handful of fresh oregano leaves

2 teaspoons onion powder

1 teaspoon garlic powder

olive oil, for greasing

1   Preheat the oven to 180°C (350°F/Gas 4).

2   For the corn crackers, bring the water and vegetable stock to the boil. Add the cornmeal, stir well, reduce the heat to low and cook to a thick mash. Stir in the oregano leaves, onion powder and garlic powder.

3   Line a baking tray with parchment paper and grease with a little bit of olive oil. Spread out the cornmeal mixture very thinly onto the prepared parchment paper and let it set and cool for a few minutes. Bake for 8–12 minutes. Turn the tray around and bake for another 6–8 minutes until evenly baked and golden brown. Take out of the oven, let it cool and turn down the oven to 150°C (300°F/Gas 2).

4   Cut the ends off the aubergines and courgettes, halve and cut into slices. Cut the tomatoes into large slices, then wash and slice the mushrooms. Line 1 or 2 baking trays with parchment paper and lay the veggies out evenly. Drizzle with olive oil and season with salt, pepper and onion powder. Sprinkle over the spring onion, garlic, chilli and oregano.

5   Fill an oven-proof dish with water and place it on the bottom of the oven. Put the vegetables into the oven and roast for 50–60 minutes.

6   Cut the spinach into small pieces, put it into a large bowl and add the remaining ingredients for the caponata. Take the roasted vegetables out of the oven, add them to the bowl and stir everything until well combined. Heat them up again if desired. The cheese should be melted and the spinach wilted.

7   Crack the cooled corn crackers into smaller pieces and serve with the caponata. A great dish where everybody can add some of the caponata to a corn cracker or enjoy it as a meal.

Tomato Couscous on a Minty Yoghurt Sauce

Sunshine on a plate.

You won't have to stand in the kitchen for very long to make this dish. The couscous is the perfect partner for the tomatoes, oriental spices and fresh ingredients like lemon, mint and pomegranate. I use quite a lot of water for the couscous in this recipe to make it nice and fluffy – just leave it to swell. With all the tasty ingredients, the couscous will be nice and moist at the end. The yoghurt sauce is also easy to make and will only take a few minutes to prepare.

––––––––––––––––––– SERVES 2 / V, RSF, DF*, VGN* –––––––––––––––––––

COUSCOUS

130–150 g (4–5 oz) wholewheat couscous
pinch of salt
250–300 ml (8½–10 fl oz) water
1–2 teaspoons coconut oil
1 spring onion (scallion), chopped
1 carrot
1 apple
1 tomato
seeds of ½ pomegranate, plus extra to serve
2 tablespoons tomato purée (paste)
zest and juice of ½ lime
½ teaspoon cumin seeds
½ teaspoon paprika powder
½ teaspoon mild or spicy curry powder
salt and freshly ground black pepper
1 teaspoon maple syrup or sweetener
   of choice
small bunch of coriander (cilantro), chopped
2 tablespoons pistachios, crushed
cress

YOGHURT SAUCE

300 g (10½ oz) natural yoghurt or *soy
   yoghurt
1 teaspoon onion powder
1 teaspoon garlic powder
½ cucumber, peeled
zest and juice of ½ lime
1 teaspoon maple syrup or sweetener
   of choice
10–15 mint leaves, chopped
drizzle of olive oil

1   Put the couscous and salt into a bowl. Bring the water to the boil, pour onto the couscous, stir, cover and leave to swell for 15–20 minutes.

2   Heat up the coconut oil in a pan. Dice the carrot, apple and tomato very finely. Fry the spring onion in the coconut oil until soft, then add the carrots and fry for another 4–5 minutes.

3   Loosen the couscous with a fork. Add the fried carrots, spring onion, diced apple and tomato, and stir. Add the remaining ingredients, except the pistachios, and stir the couscous until everything is well combined. Set aside.

4   For the sauce, put the yoghurt, garlic and onion powder into a bowl. Peel and grate the cucumber, drain the excess water, and add to the yoghurt mixture. Add the remaining ingredients except the olive oil, stir well and spread onto 2 plates.

5   Spoon the couscous on top, sprinkle with the crushed pistachios, add more pomegranate seeds and garnish with cress and a drizzle of olive oil.

TIP   You can use soy yoghurt instead of natural yoghurt in the sauce for a dairy-free and vegan version.

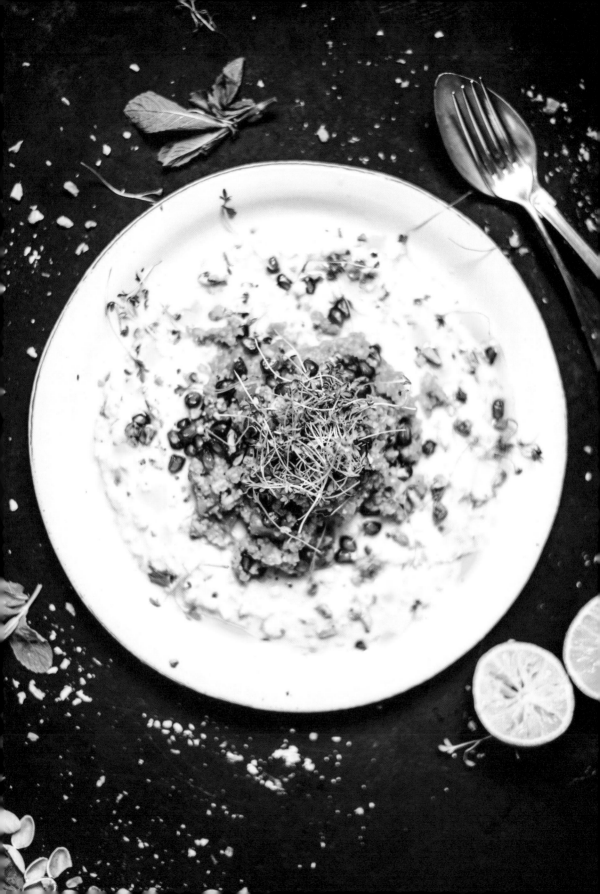

My Favourite Spinach Salad with Creamy Peanut Soy Dressing

This salad is always a winner!

A good salad dressing does wonders to a salad – more than you can imagine.
I love to come up with new dressings that are creamy and full of flavour but at the same time healthy and made with fresh ingredients. The combination of peanut butter and soy sauce simply has something magical about it. The dressing contains a fair amount of peanut butter, but doesn't contain any additional oil. To express its full flavours, it's important to add the dressing to the salad before serving it and stir until well combined. Every spinach leaf needs to be coated. Also, adding some fresh fruit – mango in this case – enhances every salad. The avocado provides extra creaminess and the honey-caramelised pecans with shredded coconut make this dish perfect and give it the crunch it needs.

—————— SERVES 2-3 / GF*, DF, V, VGN, RSF ——————

CARAMELISED PECANS

2 tablespoons crushed pecans

2 teaspoons honey

shredded coconut

SPINACH SALAD

400 g (14 oz) spinach

1 ripe mango

4–5 tablespoons fresh or frozen and thawed edamame

1 ripe avocado

40–50 g cooked quinoa per person (optional)

hemp hearts, to serve

PEANUT SOY DRESSING

1½ tablespoons peanut butter

1½ tablespoons soy sauce or *tamari

2 teaspoons maple syrup or sweetener of choice

salt and freshly ground black pepper

2 tablespoons milk of choice, e.g. soy, almond, rice milk

1 teaspoon lemon juice

1   For the caramelised pecans, put the crushed pecans, honey and shredded coconut into a frying pan (skillet), stir well and caramelise over a medium heat for 4–5 minutes. Take off the heat and let it cool completely.

2   To make the salad, wash the spinach, dry with kitchen towel or using a salad spinner and put into a large bowl.

3   Peel the mango, cut the flesh off the stone, cut into small pieces and add to the salad along with the edamame. Slice the avocado in half, remove the stone, cut half of it into small pieces, then add it to the salad. Slice the other half for the garnish and set aside.

4   For the dressing, add all the ingredients into a food processor and blend to a smooth and creamy consistency.

5   Pour the dressing over the salad and stir until well combined. If you decide to add some cooked quinoa, mix it with the salad now. Spoon onto plates.

6   Sprinkle the pecans on top of the salad, arrange the avocado slices nicely on top of the salad and finish off by sprinkling some hemp hearts on top.

VARIATIONS   If you want to add a portion of protein, I can highly recommend adding some grilled shrimp.

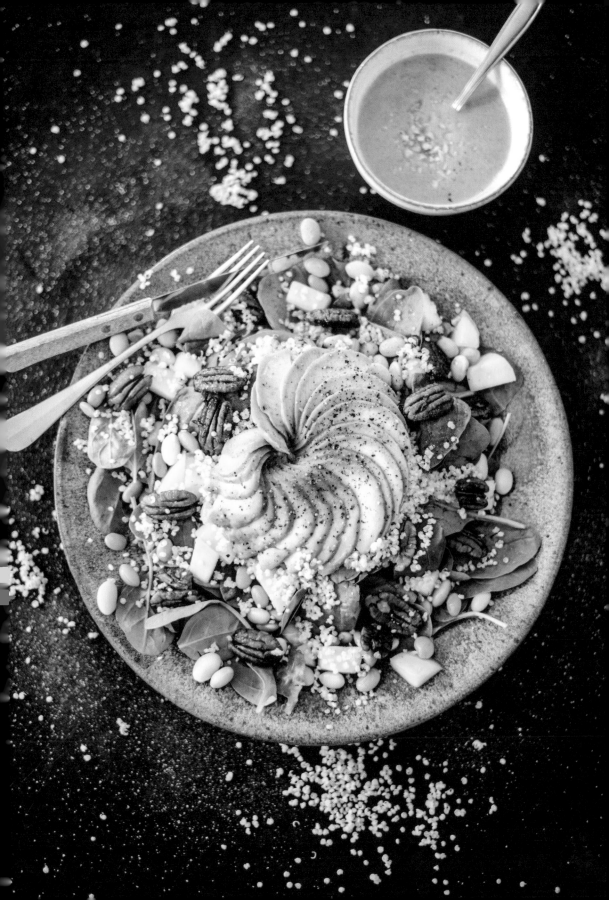

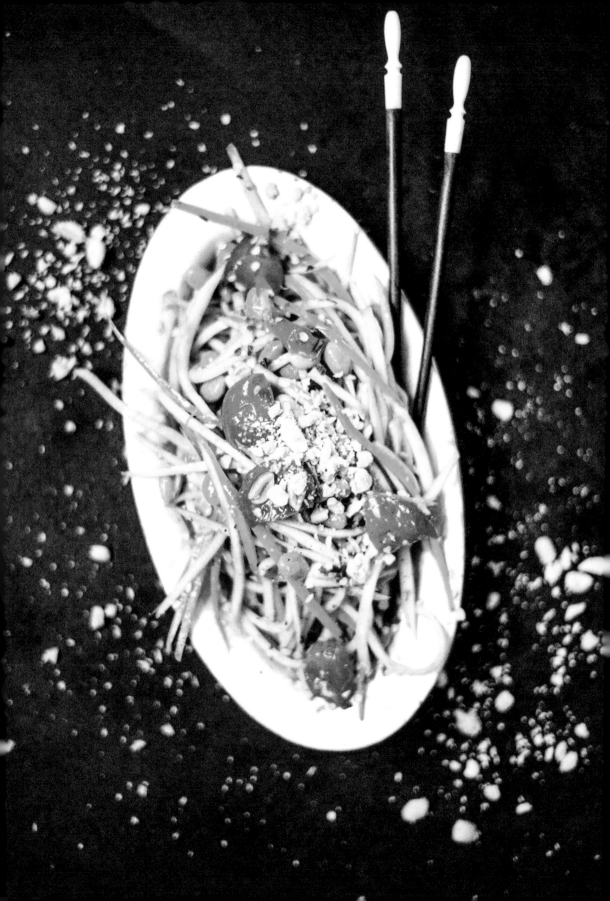

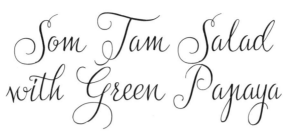

Som Tam Salad with Green Papaya

Refreshing and delicious!

If you've been to Thailand before, I'm sure you must have tried this salad. When I was travelling around Thailand, I ate this almost every day. It's the best dish to eat for lunch when it's hot outside. The main ingredients for som tam are green papaya, tomatoes, long beans, peanuts, dried shrimp and a very easy dressing. I have replaced some ingredients and added others to give it my personal touch. But all in all, it tastes very similar. And anyone who wants to try the original – hop on the next flight and make a trip to Thailand right away!

SERVES 2 / V, DF

SALAD

1 garlic clove, finely chopped

½ red chilli

1 spring onion (scallion)

3 tablespoons peanuts

12–15 cherry tomatoes

4 tablespoons edamame

250–300 g (9–10½ oz) green papaya

1 carrot

handful of beansprouts

DRESSING

2 tablespoons fish sauce

1 tablespoon oyster sauce

juice of 1 lime

salt and freshly ground black pepper

2–3 teaspoons maple syrup or sweetener of choice

1   Put the garlic and chilli into a mortar. The more chilli seeds you add, the spicier it will be. Chop the spring onion and add to the mortar together with 2 tablespoons of the peanuts. Crush in the mortar and pestle for a few minutes, then transfer into a bowl. Cut the cherry tomatoes in half and put them with the edamame into the mortar and pestle. Crush again for about a minute, then add them to the bowl too.

2   Peel the papaya, cut it in half and remove the seeds. Peel the carrot and cut off the ends. Cut both the papaya and carrot into long strips with a julienne peeler. Add to the tomato and edamame mixture along with the beansprouts and mix well until combined.

3   In a bowl, stir together all the ingredients for the dressing. Pour over the salad and mix well. Taste and decide for yourself whether you'd like to add more lime juice, maple syrup, fish sauce or oyster sauce.

4   Divide the salad into bowls. Crush the remaining peanuts and sprinkle on top.

GREEN PAPAYA   You can get green papaya at almost every Asian store all year round. If you can't find any at all though, replace it with 1 white radish and 1–2 unripe pears and prepare the same way. It won't quite taste the same, but it's still very delicious!

Roasted Corn on the Cob with Garlic & Rosemary Hummus

A little extra garlic never hurt anybody!

Sometimes you just need a lot of garlic! But why is something we all love something we reject so often? I know, I know, it's the smell afterwards. I have this love-hate relationship as well, but it's about 99 percent love. Whenever there's garlic in a dish, it simply tastes a bit better. With this dish, every garlic lover, corn lover and vegetarian will be able to satisfy his or her taste buds.

SERVES 2 / GF, V, RSF

CORNS

2 sweetcorn cobs

2 teaspoons coconut oil, melted

sea salt

HUMMUS

250 g (9 oz) chickpeas (garbanzos), cooked or soaked

salt and freshly ground black pepper

1 teaspoon garlic powder

2–4 garlic cloves

5 sprigs of fresh rosemary

2 teaspoons tahini

1 tablespoon olive oil

salt and freshly ground black pepper

zest and juice of 1 lemon

4 tablespoons Greek or *soy yoghurt

drizzle of honey

1   Preheat the oven to 180°C (350°F/Gas 4). Line a baking tray with parchment paper.

2   For the hummus, drain the chickpeas and season with salt, pepper and garlic powder. Tip them onto the baking tray. Peel and halve the garlic cloves and lay around the chickpeas along with 4 sprigs of the rosemary. Roast for 15–20 minutes. Take the chickpeas out of the oven and put them into the food processor with the roasted garlic and rosemary.

3   Add the remaining ingredients, except the honey, to the food processor. Blend for at least 4–5 minutes until smooth and creamy. Spoon into a bowl, drizzle some honey on top and garnish with the remaining rosemary.

4   Preheat the oven to 200°C (400°F/Gas 6).

5   Remove any husks from the corn and rub with the melted coconut oil. Season with sea salt and wrap each corn cob in foil. Bake for 40 minutes.

6   Take the roasted corn out of the oven, cut each cob into 3 pieces and spread some of the hummus on top. For the full flavour, cut the corn off the stalks, add into a bowl, spoon in a few tablespoons of the hummus and stir until well combined.

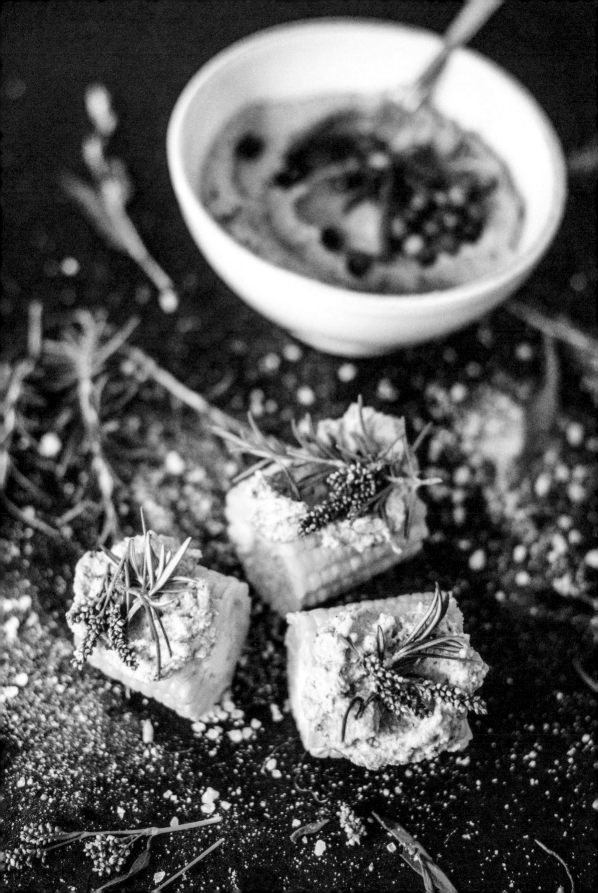

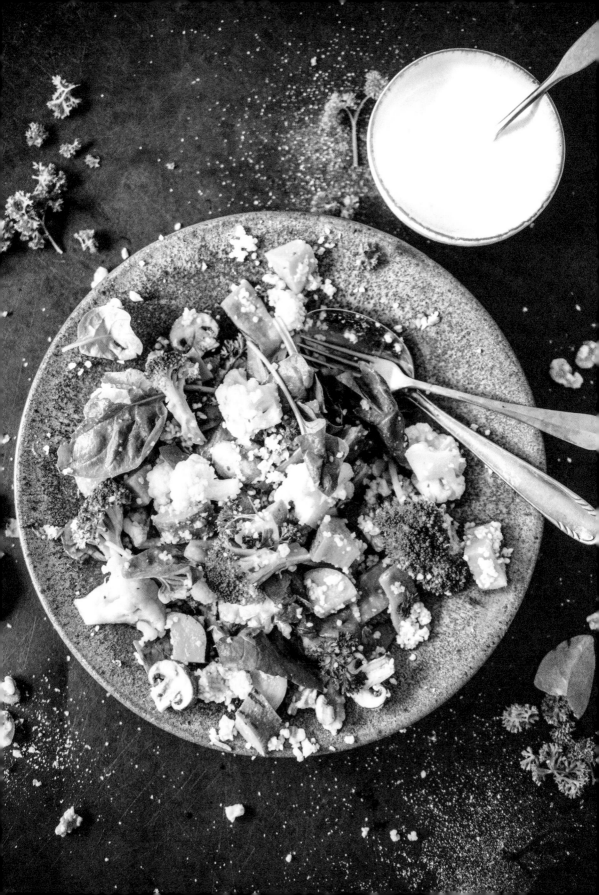

Colourful Vegetables & Millet with Silken Tofu Dip

Great to fill your lunch box!

Whenever you don't have a lot of time and want to bring something with you for lunch, this is the right dish for you. It's filled with good nutrients, vegetables and greens and contains good carbs to keep you full and energised for a few hours. The vegetables are best when you don't fry them for too long so that they stay crunchy. The smooth and creamy dip goes along very well with every kind of vegetable. Furthermore, millet is one of my favourite grains. If you cook it a few extra minutes, it gets even creamier.

SERVES 2 / GF, DF, V, VGN, RSF

MILLET & VEGETABLES

1 medium sweet potato

6 tablespoons millet

1 teaspoon coconut oil or olive oil

½ teaspoon salt

1 teaspoon vegetable broth

150 ml (5 fl oz) water

150 g (5 oz) broccoli

150 g (5 oz) cauliflower

150 g (5 oz) green beans

150 g (5 oz) button mushrooms

bunch of fresh parsley

2 handfuls of spinach

lemon juice, to serve

8–10 walnuts, crushed, to serve

parsley, to garnish

TOFU DIP

250 g (9 oz) silken tofu

zest and juice of 1 lemon

40–50 g (1½–2 oz) cashews

1 teaspoon onion powder

1 teaspoon garlic powder

1 teaspoon maple syrup or sweetener of choice

salt and freshly ground black pepper

1   For the dip, put all the ingredients into a blender and blend to a smooth and creamy consistency for 4–5 minutes.

2   Peel the sweet potato and dice into approximately 1 cm (½ in) cubes. Put the sweet potato into a saucepan of water and bring to the boil along with the millet, oil and salt and cook over a medium heat for 5–7 minutes. Remove from the heat and allow the millet to swell for about 10 minutes. Drain and transfer to a large bowl.

3   Bring another saucepan of water to the boil with the vegetable stock. Cut the broccoli and cauliflower off the stalk and tear into florets. Slice the mushrooms, then cut the ends off the beans and halve. Put the broccoli, cauliflower, mushrooms, beans and parsley into the pan and cook over a medium heat for a few minutes, making sure that the vegetables stay crisp. Add the spinach at the last minute to soften slightly. Drain and add to the sweet potato and millet.

4   Stir half of the dip into the vegetables and serve the other half as a dip on the side for those who want to add some more. Divide onto plates, squeeze over some lemon juice and sprinkle the walnuts and some parsley on top.

Superfood Tricolore Salad

Provides you with so much energy!

A flavour and energy bomb all in one, this is my favourite salad to have either after a workout or for brunch. I'll admit, it's more time consuming to make than other salads, but it's time well-invested because I'm sure you're going to love it. You can cook three to four times the amount of quinoa and keep it in the fridge to use for other dishes. Quinoa is gluten-free and very high in protein, keeps you full and, with the right spices, it's so tasty! This is a real superfood salad with a refreshing lemon and tahini dressing for an extra portion of energy.

SERVES 1 OR 2 AS A STARTER / GF, DF, V, VGN*, RSF

SALAD

200–250 g (7–9 oz) kale

50 g (2 oz) tricolore quinoa

pinch of salt

150 ml (5 fl oz) water

1 courgette (zucchini)

coconut oil, for frying

1 tablespoon flaked (slivered) almonds

½ avocado, sliced

1 egg *(optional)

1 tablespoon white wine vinegar (optional)

2 teaspoons hemp seeds

cress, to garnish

DRESSING

1½ tablespoons lemon juice

1½ tablespoons white wine vinegar

1 tablespoon olive oil

2 teaspoons tahini

salt and freshly ground black pepper

1–2 teaspoons maple syrup or sweetener of choice

1   Remove the kale leaves from the stalks, tear into smaller pieces, wash, dry well with a salad spinner and put into a bowl.

2   For the dressing, whisk all the ingredients in a bowl until well combined. Pour over the kale and massage the dressing into the leaves for at least 3–4 minutes until the tough kale has wilted slightly without losing its bite.

3   Bring the water, salt and quinoa to the boil and cook over a medium heat for about 12–15 minutes until the water has evaporated. Take off the heat and leave to cool.

4   Slice the courgette. Heat some coconut oil in a frying pan (skillet) and fry the courgette for a few minutes until golden brown. Toast the almonds in a dry frying pan over a medium heat until golden brown. Take off the heat and leave to cool.

5   Add the quinoa and courgette to the kale salad, stir again, and transfer onto a plate. Top with avocado slices and garnish with the toasted almonds.

6   If you want to add a poached egg on top as well for some more protein, bring 500 ml (17 fl oz) of water to a boil, reduce the heat to a simmer, add the white wine vinegar, stir the water with a whisk until it is swirling, crack the egg and carefully slide it into the centre of the pan. After 2–3 minutes, when the egg white is cooked but the yolk is still soft, use a slotted spoon to take the egg out of the water. Remove any excess water with kitchen towel and place the poached egg on top of the salad.

7   Sprinkle the hemp seeds on top, garnish with cress and serve.

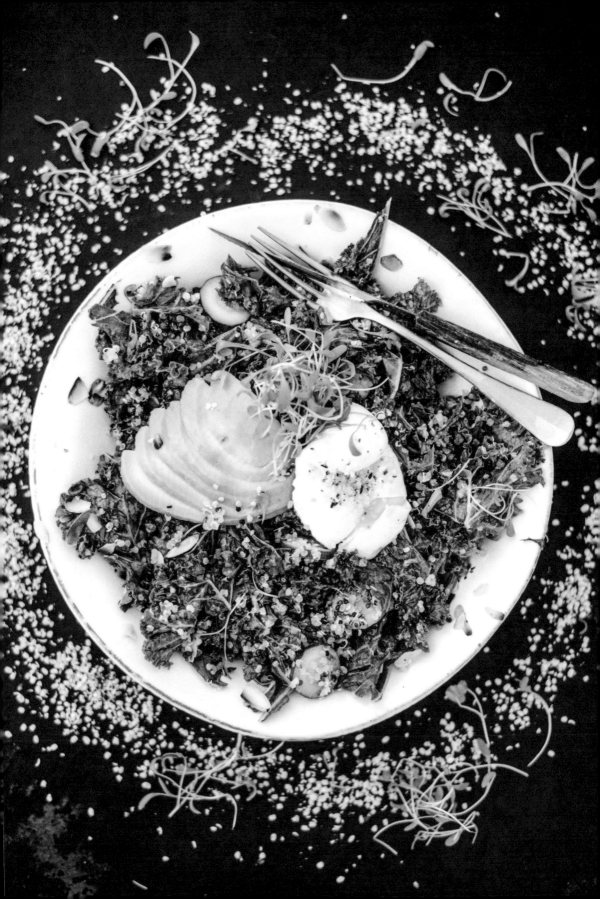

Sweet Potato & Vegetable Crisps with Guacamole

Healthy crisps (chips) and heavenly avocado dip: goodbye deep-fried crisps!
Don't we all know it and fall for it every once in a while? We're sitting in front of the TV and get bored. Until we come up with the great idea of having a bag of crisps.
Not such a great idea, actually, because store-bought crisps are, almost without exception, deep-fried, and contain sugar and many other preservatives. I created a recipe for you so that you can enjoy eating crisps, plus a healthy dip, without feeling guilty at all.
They're free from oil and preservatives, super crunchy and have something for everybody!

SERVES 3-4 (AS A SNACK) / GF, *DF, V, *VGN, RSF

CRISPS (CHIPS)

1 medium sweet potato

1 large carrot

2 beetroots (beets)

1 parsnip

1 teaspoon onion powder

salt and freshly ground black pepper

DIP

1 avocado

zest and juice of 1 lime

1 teaspoon ground coriander (cilantro)

salt and freshly ground black pepper

1 teaspoon garlic powder

1 teaspoon onion powder

drizzle of honey

2–3 tablespoons *soy yoghurt or yoghurt of choice

1   Preheat the oven to 170°C (340°F/Gas 3½). Line 2 baking trays with parchment paper.

2   To make the crisps, peel the vegetables and slice them very thinly. Lay them out evenly on the prepared baking tray and season with onion powder, salt and pepper. Bake for 35–45 minutes until golden brown and crispy. Always keep an eye on them, as depending on how evenly you sliced the vegetables some crisps might be done before others. To perform a 'crunch test', take a golden-brown baked crisp out of the oven, let it cool for a bit and try it. If it's crunchy then they're good, otherwise leave them in the oven for a few more minutes.

3   For the avocado dip, cut the avocado in half, remove the stone, peel and add the flesh into a bowl. Add all the other ingredients for the dip into the bowl and mash with a fork until well combined. Don't blend the dip – it's so much better when it's still a little bit chunky.

4   If you haven't already, remove the crisps from the oven and let them cool for at least 5 minutes. Serve with the avocado dip.

VARIATIONS   For those of you who like it hot just like me, add some chilli powder to the avocado dip. (This is also a good idea if you want the whole dip for yourself because you are the only one who likes it hot!)

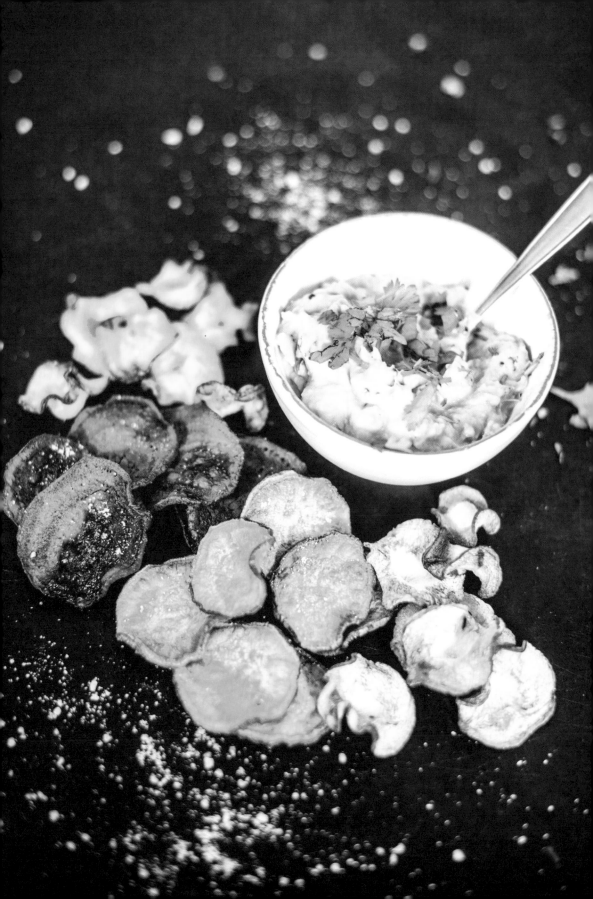

Vietnamese Shrimp Rolls with Orange & Lime Dressing

More refreshing and less oily than fried spring rolls.
These rolls are perfect to serve in summer. For the vegetarian and vegan versions,
make them without the shrimp or replace with tofu or another vegetable of choice.

SERVES 2 (3-4 AS A STARTER) / *GF, DF, RSF

RICE PAPER ROLLS

8 large rice paper sheets

2 tablespoons water

2–3 teaspoons *tamari or soy sauce

1 teaspoon honey

2 carrots, thinly sliced

100 g (3½ oz) beansprouts

1 teaspoon coconut oil

1 spring onion (scallion), chopped

18–24 fresh prawns (shrimp)

1 ripe avocado

4–6 tablespoons edamame

sea salt

½ mango

2–3 handfuls of fresh spinach

DRESSING

zest and juice of 1 orange

zest and juice of ½ lime

2 tablespoons white balsamic vinegar

1 tablespoon olive oil

2–3 teaspoons maple syrup or
   sweetener of choice

10–15 mint leaves

1 teaspoon onion powder

salt and freshly ground black pepper

1   For the rice paper rolls, heat up the water, tamari and honey in a frying pan (skillet) over a medium–high heat. Add the carrots and beansprouts and cook for 2–3 minutes. The vegetables should remain slightly crispy. Take off the heat and put into a bowl.

2   Heat up the coconut oil in another frying pan and fry the spring onion until golden brown. Add the prawns and fry for another few minutes, then take off the heat and set aside.

3   Cut the avocado in half, remove the stone, peel and cut into thin slices. Peel the mango, cut the flesh off the stone and cut into thin slices as well. Season the edamame with sea salt.

4   Add all the ingredients for the dressing into a food processor and blend for 2–3 minutes until it foams up a little.

5   Start making the rolls one by one. Fill a large pan with warm water. Soak one rice paper sheet in the water for about 10 seconds, take out and place onto the kitchen surface. On the bottom two thirds, leaving space at the edges, add 2 slices each of mango and avocado. Then add some spinach and edamame, a spoonful of the cooked vegetables and 3 prawns. Drizzle some dressing on top.

6   Fold in the bottom of the rice paper, tuck in the sides and roll up tight. Repeat with the remaining rice paper sheets until you have no more filling left. Serve with the remaining dressing to drizzle on top. Make sure not to add too much filling to the rolls because the sheets can tear very easily if overfilled.

TIP   Double the recipe for the dressing, add 2 tablespoons of soy yoghurt or other yoghurt of choice, 2 teaspoons of almond butter, another drizzle of lime juice and serve as dipping sauce.

VARIATIONS   If you're really hungry: put a good handful of cooked glass noodles into a bowl, add 2–3 teaspoons of both fish and oyster sauce, some chilli, lime juice and a drizzle of maple syrup, stir well and spoon more on top of the spinach before adding the prawns, then roll up.

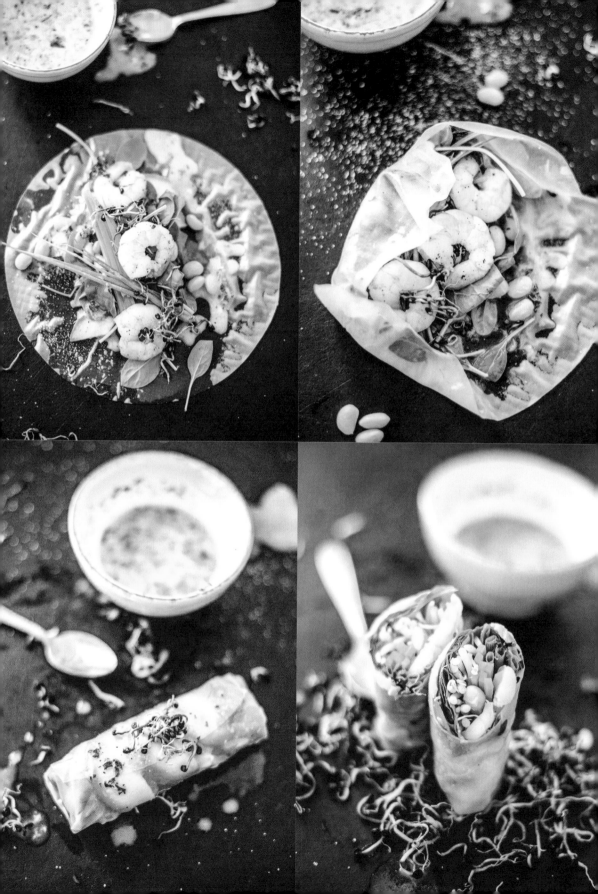

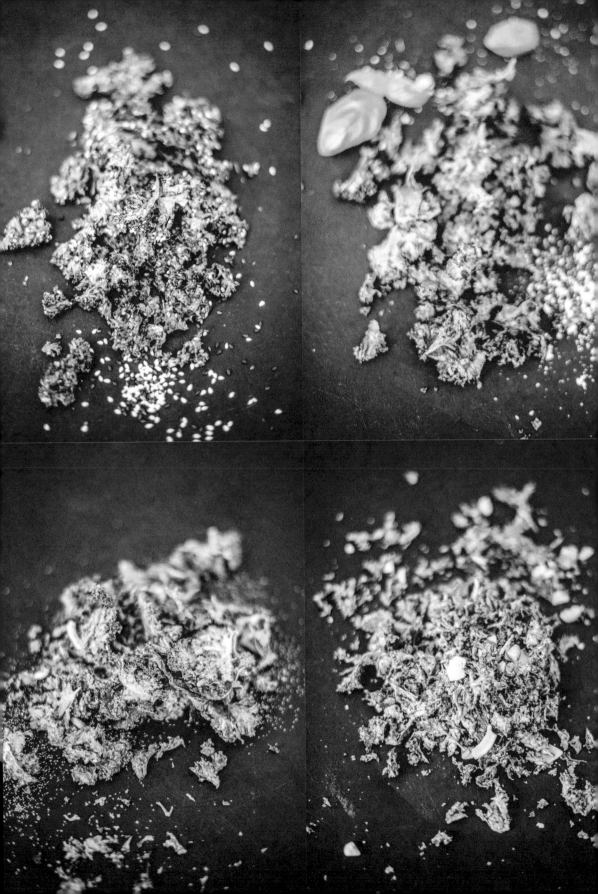

Baked Kale Crisps Four Ways

Kale makes it possible!
They're light, crunchy and so incredibly tasty. Your first thought might be, 'What?!
Crisps (chips) made out of salad?!' I had exactly the same thought until I tried a few
different kale crisp variations. Now I'm obsessed and can't resist them. I mean, who can
say no to tasty and healthy crisps?

SERVES 2-3 / *GF, V, RSF

350 g (12 oz) kale leaves

THE ORIGINAL

2–3 tablespoons olive oil

1 teaspoon sea salt and freshly ground black
  pepper

SOUR CREAM & ONION

50 g (2 oz) cashews, soaked in water for
  1–2 hours or overnight

2 tablespoons lemon juice

1 tablespoon apple cider vinegar

2–3 teaspoons onion powder

1 teaspoon garlic powder

salt and freshly ground black pepper

1 tablespoon water

ASIAN

2 tablespoons *tamari or soy sauce

½ tablespoon peanut butter

2–3 teaspoons honey

1 tablespoon sesame seeds

CAPRESE

2 tablespoons tomato purée (paste)

2 tablespoons grated Parmesan

½ tablespoons dried basil

salt and freshly ground black pepper

balsamic glaze

CURRY NUTS

2 tablespoons peanut butter

1–2 tablespoons unsweetened coconut chips

1 teaspoon maple syrup

1 teaspoon curry powder

sea salt

1   Preheat the oven to 150°C (300°F/Gas 2). Line 2 baking trays with parchment paper.

2   Remove the kale leaves from the stalks and tear, if necessary, into LARGE pieces. Wash and dry really well in a salad spinner, add into a large bowl.

FOR THE ORIGINAL   Drizzle the olive oil on top, season with salt and pepper and massage the kale leaves for 2–3 minutes until they are soft. Lay out in a single layer on the baking trays and bake for about 20–30 minutes, until they are slightly browned. Remove from the oven and let them cool completely so that they can get crunchy, then serve.

FOR THE SOUR CREAM & ONION   Put all the ingredients into a blender or food processor and blend for 4–6 minutes to a smooth and creamy consistency, comparable to a thick salad dressing. Pour the mixture over the kale leaves and massage until the leaves are completely covered with the dressing. Lay them out on the prepared baking trays in a single layer and bake for 15–25 minutes until golden brown. Take out of the oven, let them cool completely and serve.

FOR THE OTHER FLAVOURS   Mix all the ingredients together and massage into the kale leaves with your hands for a few minutes until the leaves are covered. Lay them out on the prepared baking trays in a single layer and bake for 15–25 minutes until slightly browned. Take out of the oven, let them cool completely and serve.

TIP   Always keep an eye on the crisps because they can easily burn. The baking times can vary depending on how tough the kale leaves are and depending on the dressing. To check it they're ready, simply take one crisp out of the oven, let it cool quickly and give it a try to see if it's crunchy.

Sweet Potato Fries with Heavenly Tahini Dip

This dip makes you completely forget about mayo.

Who said you can't eat fries as part of a healthy diet? This recipe proves that you can. They're a little different, but just as good – if not better. But what's different? First of all, I use sweet potato instead of regular potatoes. They are lower in calories and higher in fibre. Also, these fries are baked and not fried. Unlike mayo and ketchup, this tahini dip doesn't contain any refined sugar or preservatives. It contains healthy fats from the nut butter and tahini and no preservatives at all. Plus, it delivers so much more taste and freshness. These sweet potato fries are great to serve as an appetiser with the tahini dip, which is also a tasty dip for vegetable sticks.

SERVES 2-3 / GF, *DF, V, *VGN, RSF

SWEET POTATO FRIES

3 medium sweet potatoes

1 tablespoon olive oil

½ teaspoon paprika

½ teaspoon onion powder

salt and freshly ground black pepper

2–3 sprigs parsley or thyme, to garnish

TAHINI DIP

4 tablespoons natural yoghurt or
   *soy yoghurt

1½ tablespoons tahini

1 tablespoon lemon juice

1 teaspoon peanut butter

6–8 cashews

2 teaspoons maple syrup or sweetener
   of choice

salt and freshly ground black pepper

1 teaspoon garlic powder

1 teaspoon onion powder

splash of milk of choice, e.g. soy, almond,
   rice milk (optional)

1   Preheat the oven to 200°C (400°F/Gas 6). Line 2 baking trays with parchment paper.

2   To make the fries, cut the ends off the sweet potatoes, peel and cut into matchsticks. Put them into a large bowl, drizzle the olive oil on top, add all the spices and mix well with your hands.

3   Lay the sweet potato fries out on the prepared baking trays in a single layer (not on top of each other!) and bake for 25–35 minutes until golden brown. To perform the 'crunch test', take a fry out of the oven, let it cool for a bit and try it. If they're not crispy or crunchy enough, bake for a few more minutes.

4   For the tahini dip, put all the ingredients into a blender and blend to a smooth and creamy mixture. If desired, add a splash of milk of choice to make it a bit creamier. Blend again and pour into a bowl.

5   Take the sweet potato fries out of the oven, let them cool so that they can get crispy, add some chopped herbs on top and serve with the tahini dip.

VARIATIONS   You can replace the sweet potato with yam. Prepare in the same way. They even get a little crunchier after baking than the sweet potato fries.

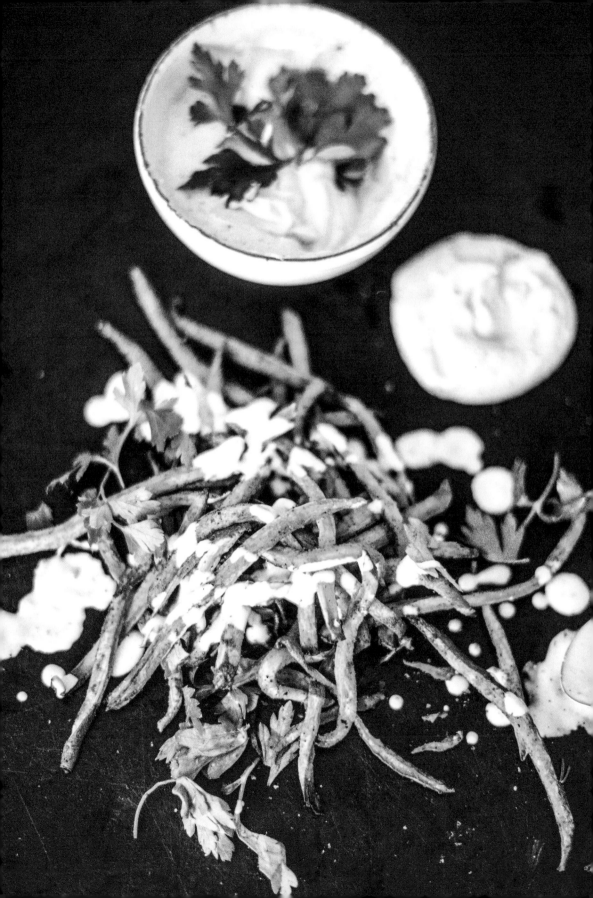

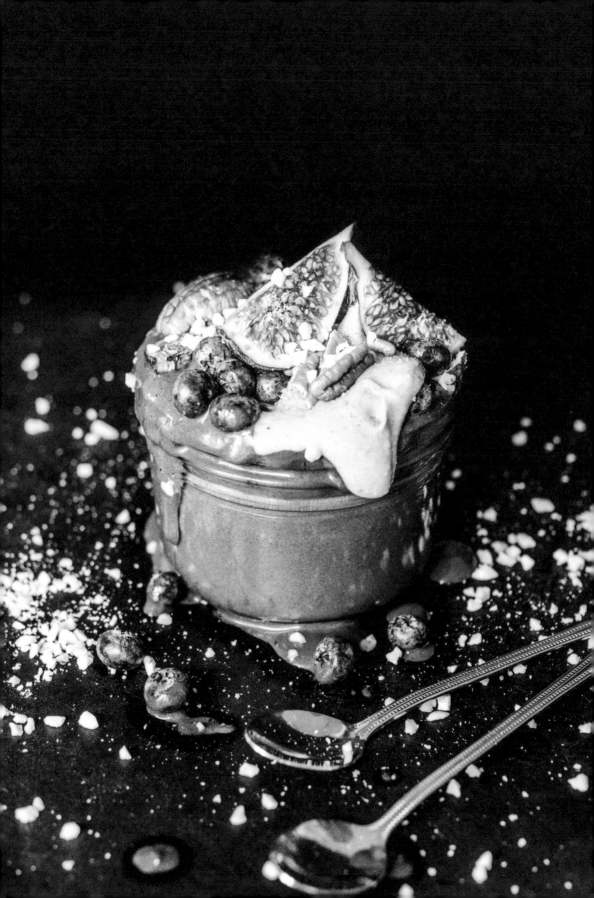

DESSERTS

Innocent & Sweet

GF= GLUTEN-FREE · DF= DAIRY-FREE

V= VEGETARIAN · VGN= VEGAN · RSF= REFINED-SUGAR-FREE

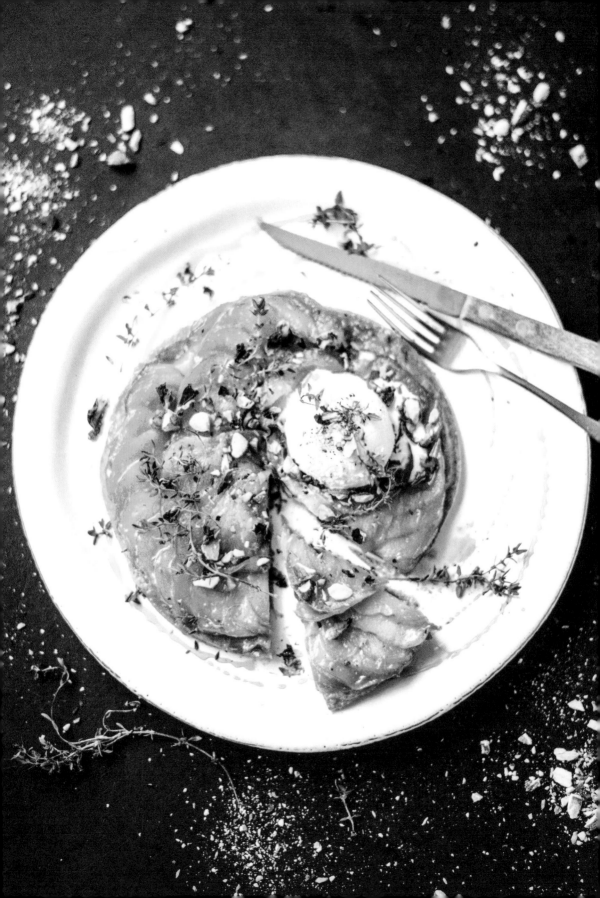

Tarte Tatin with Coconut & Thyme Ice Cream

Reinvented: the popular French tart.

Tarte tatin is a French puff pastry apple tart baked upside down, meaning that you bake the tart with the pastry on top and flip it over afterwards. In the original recipe you spread butter in a cake tin, then add some sugar on top, which caramelises. I use coconut oil and almond butter for my version, and add honey instead. I replace the puff pastry in the original with a wholewheat tortilla. The coconut and thyme ice cream gives this reinterpreted tarte tatin a refreshing kick.

SERVES 1-2 (1 CAKE TIN 20 CM (8 IN) / DF, VGN, RSF

ICE CREAM

1 banana, sliced and frozen

1 tablespoon shredded coconut

splash of coconut milk

2 teaspoons maple syrup or sweetener of choice

1 teaspoon coconut oil

1–2 sprigs of thyme, leaves picked

TART

2 teaspoons coconut oil, melted

2 teaspoons almond butter

2 teaspoons maple syrup or sweetener of choice, plus extra to serve

pinch of salt

1 vanilla bean, seeds scraped

1–2 sprigs of thyme, leaves picked, plus extra sprigs to garnish

1–2 small apples

1 wholewheat tortilla

roasted and crushed almonds or nuts of choice, to serve

1   Preheat the oven to 180°C (350°F/Gas 4).

2   For the ice cream, take the frozen banana out of the freezer and allow to thaw for a few minutes. Add the banana and remaining ingredients to a food processor and blend until smooth. Spoon into a container and put back into the freezer.

3   To make the tart, spread the melted coconut oil into the cake tin. Mix the almond butter with the maple syrup, salt and vanilla seeds and add to the cake tin as well. Add the thyme leaves on top and smooth out the mixture evenly.

4   Cut the apples into quarters, remove the cores and cut them into very thin slices. Layer the slices in the cake tin, creating a circle from the outside to the centre of the tin. Bake for 8–10 minutes.

5   Take the tin out of the oven, put the tortilla onto the apples and press down a little. Turn down the oven to 160°C (320°F/Gas 2) and bake for another 6–8 minutes until the tortilla has browned.

6   Remove the tin from the oven and flip it upside down on to a plate. The tart should slide out of the tin easily.

7   Take the ice cream out of the freezer and add 1–2 scoops onto the warm tortilla. Garnish with thyme and almonds, and drizzle some maple syrup on top. Enjoy right away!

Home-made Chocolate Your Favourite Way

Also makes a great gift.

Dark chocolate has quite a high cocoa content. It's proven to be good for your heart as well as for your psyche and it contains minerals as well as plenty of antioxidants. When I buy dark chocolate, I like to get chocolate with a high cocoa content, around 70 percent. For this recipe, you can buy a dark chocolate with a cocoa content starting from 70 percent up to as high as you like. The only other things you need are your favourite nutritious toppings and a pinch of creativity!

1 CHOCOLATE BAR/ GF, DF, VGN, RSF*

50–70 g (2–2½ oz) min. 70% cocoa dark chocolate, or *dark chocolate sweetened with stevia

PISTACHIO & CRANBERRY

2 tablespoons pistachios, roasted and crushed

1 tablespoon shredded coconut

1 tablespoon dried unsweetened cranberries

HAZELNUT & MULBERRY

2 tablespoons hazelnuts, roasted

1 tablespoon dried mulberries

ALMOND & POMEGRANATE

1 tablespoon flaked (slivered) almonds

1 tablespoon Sesame Coconut Chips (see page 96)

1 tablespoon dried pomegranate seeds

PEANUT & CASHEW

1 tablespoon peanut butter

1 teaspoon sweetener of choice, preferably maple syrup

½ tablespoon crushed cashews

1   Cut some parchment paper into rectangular pieces about 15 × 25 cm (6 × 8 in) (cut more or fewer depending on how many bars you're making) and lay them out on the work surface.

2   Break the chocolate into smaller pieces and melt in a small heatproof bowl sat over a saucepan of hot water.

3   Pour the melted chocolate onto the prepared pieces of parchment paper, spread it out into a rectangular chocolate bar and add the toppings of your choice. Freeze for at least two hours.

4   Take the chocolate out of the freezer and break into pieces. Enjoy a piece as a little dessert after a meal or to satisfy your sweet cravings.

STORAGE   Leave the chocolate in a suitable container in the freezer; it stays firm and you can keep it for longer. When it's too cold for you to eat right out of the freezer, put some pieces into the fridge to thaw for a few minutes and then enjoy.

*CHOCOLATE   You can find chocolate sweetened with stevia at health food stores. If you don't like the taste of stevia, choose a chocolate sweetened with coconut sugar or raw cane sugar for this recipe instead.

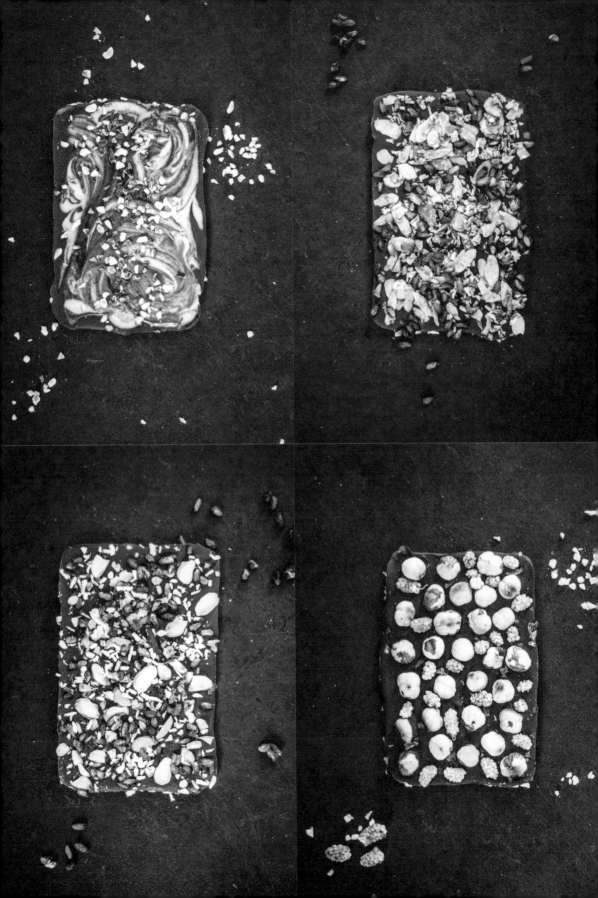

Banana Sushi

Turns everybody into a real sushi fan.

When it comes to sushi, preferences are usually extreme. Some could eat it daily, others have tried it once and it stops there. I'm sure that everybody who has a weakness for sweet things like chocolate and loves bananas will turn into a sweet sushi lover in no time. The taste can't be compared with 'proper' sushi, but you can also eat it with chopsticks and it even comes with a 'soy sauce' for dipping. A sweet and healthy treat that will blow your taste buds away.

MAKES 1 ROLL/6-8 PIECES / DF, VGN, RSF

BANANA SUSHI

1 wholewheat tortilla

2–3 teaspoons Chocolate & Hazelnut Butter (see page 36) or nut butter of choice

1 ripe banana

finely crushed nuts of choice, to serve

SAUCE

150 g (5 oz) fresh or frozen and thawed raspberries and strawberries or berries of choice

1 teaspoon maple syrup or sweetener of choice

1 Put the wholewheat tortilla on to a plate and spread the nut butter over two thirds of the tortilla.

2 Add the banana on top and roll the tortilla up tight.

3 For the sauce, cook the berries together with the sweetener until soft. Then either blend quickly or mash up with a fork.

4 Heat a frying pan over a medium heat, then toast the sushi roll on all sides until golden brown. Remove from the heat and allow to cool slightly.

5 Cut the sushi roll into 1–2 cm (½–¾ in) thick slices, put them onto a plate, sprinkle some finely crushed nuts on top and serve with the berry sauce.

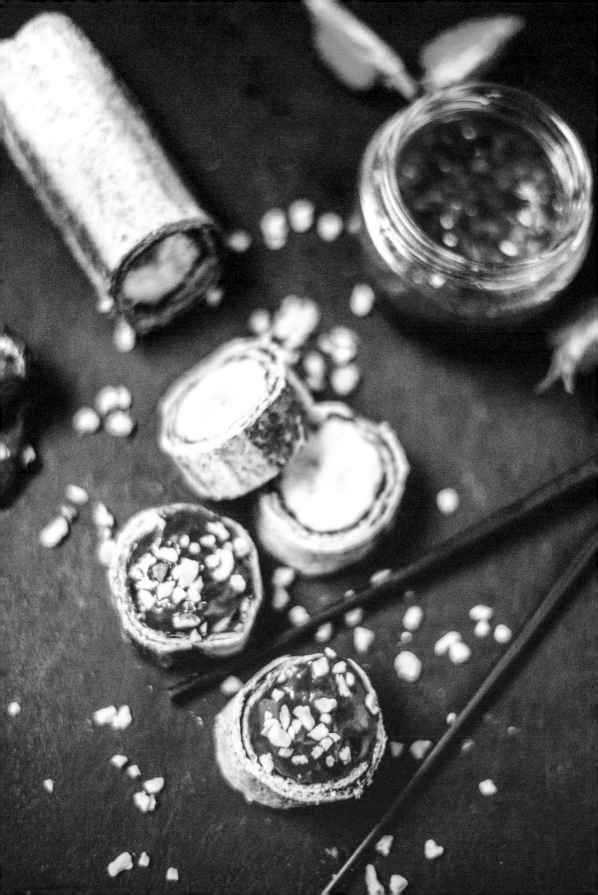

Deliciously Tempting
Chocolate Mousse & Peanut Cream

A must-try for dessert lovers!

A healthy chocolate mousse made with avocado and a peanut cream made out of sweet potato. Doesn't sound good? Then you should run into your kitchen right now and give it a try. Both desserts will lead you into a completely new world of how different yet tasty desserts can be, with ingredients you normally wouldn't think of using. Two recipes that are not only super easy to make, but also make you want to lick the bowl clean. And if you can't decide which one to try first, simply make them both!

SERVES 2 EACH / GF, DF, VGN, RSF

CHOCOLATE MOUSSE

2 Medjool dates or 4 small dates, pitted

½ ripe avocado

1 ripe banana,

2 tablespoons raw cacao powder

2–3 teaspoons maple syrup or sweetener of choice

pinch of salt

dash of milk of choice, e.g. soy, almond, rice milk

PEANUT CREAM

½ medium sweet potato

4 Medjool dates or 8 small dates, pitted

2 tablespoons peanut butter

2–3 teaspoons maple syrup, or sweetener of choice

250 ml (8½ fl oz) milk of choice, e.g. soy, almond, rice milk

1 vanilla bean, seeds scraped scraepd

TOPPINGS

fruits and berries of choice

nuts of choice, roasted and crushed

1   For the chocolate mousse, soak the dates in boiling water for 5–10 minutes.

2   Cut the avocado in half, remove the stone and put the flesh into a food processor. Drain the dates and add to the avocado. Add the rest of the ingredients except the milk and blend everything until smooth and creamy. Depending on the consistency, you might have to add a splash of milk to make the chocolate mousse creamier.

3   Spoon into small bowls and chill in the fridge for 1–2 hours to set.

4   For the peanut cream, cut the ends off the sweet potato, peel and cut into smaller pieces. In a medium-sized saucepan, bring some water to the boil, add the sweet potato and dates, and cook for about 15 minutes until soft. Drain, add to a food processor with the remaining ingredients and blend to a smooth consistency.

5   Spoon into small bowls and chill for 1–2 hours.

6   Top both desserts with your berries or fruit of choice and sprinkle roasted and crushed nuts on top.

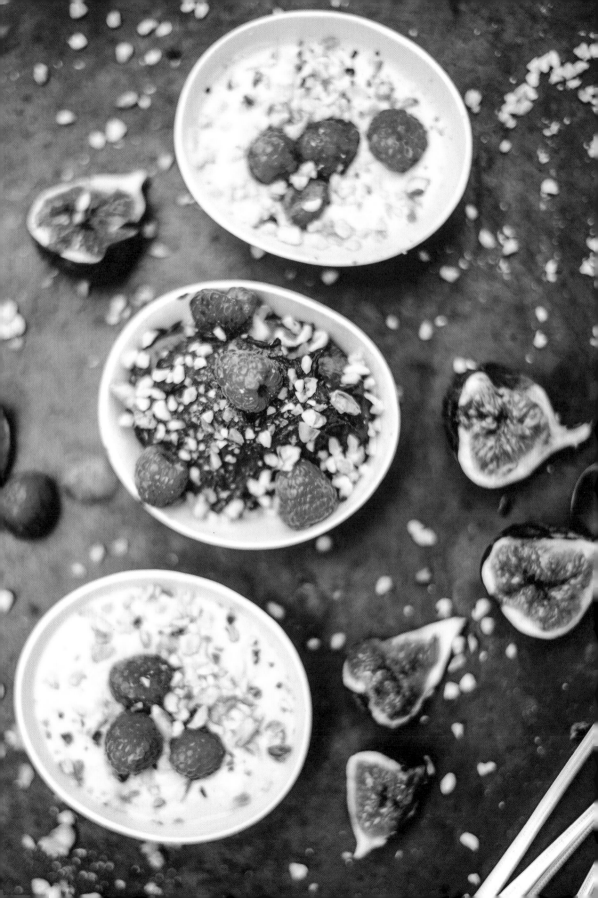

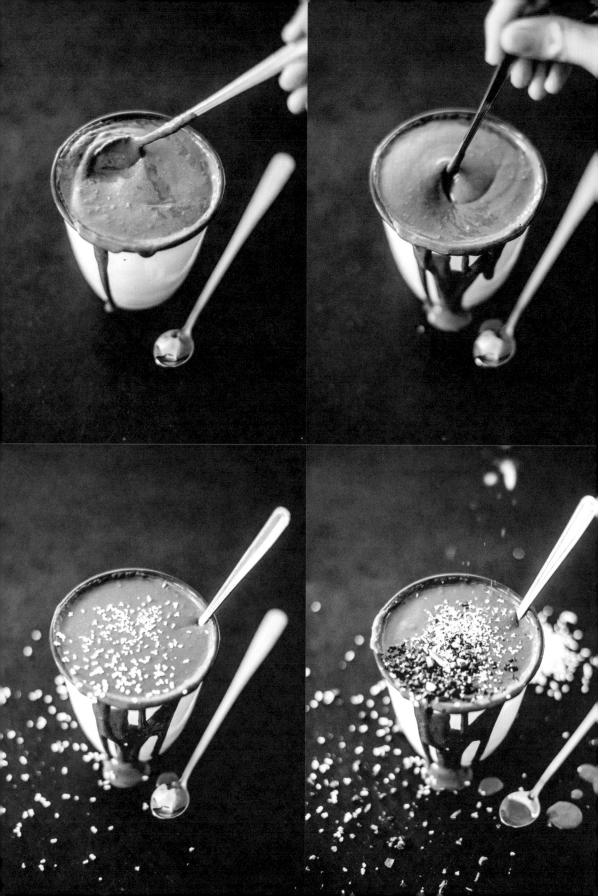

Creamy Amaranth Hot Chocolate

Outside it's getting cold, inside it's getting chocolatey.

When winter approaches, we begin to crave a hot and heart-warming drink (chocolate in my case) more and more. I personally love to spoon out everything, so I like it when the consistency of my hot chocolate is a bit thicker. My version doesn't contain any sugar, refined chocolate or lactose. I also blend in some puffed amaranth and dates to make the chocolate rich and creamy. You're free to choose any type of milk, but I prefer to use my favourites – soy milk, rice milk or almond milk.

SERVES 2 / GF, DF, VGN, RSF

300 ml (10½ oz) milk of choice, e.g. soy, almond, rice milk

200 ml (7 fl oz) water

4 tablespoons raw cacao powder

4 tablespoons puffed amaranth

4 Medjool dates

1 tablespoon maple syrup or sweetener of choice

1   Put all the ingredients into a large saucepan, bring to the boil and cook on a medium–low heat for about 10–12 minutes. Stir from time to time.

2   Take the pan off the heat and blend until creamy with a hand blender for at least 2–3 minutes. The longer you blend, the creamier the hot chocolate gets. Pour into cups and serve with your favourite spoon.

TIP   If you're not the biggest fan of hot chocolate but you like chocolate in general, make this recipe the same way but let the hot chocolate cool completely in the fridge for a few hours. The cooled hot chocolate can also be eaten with a spoon like a chocolate cream – super tasty!

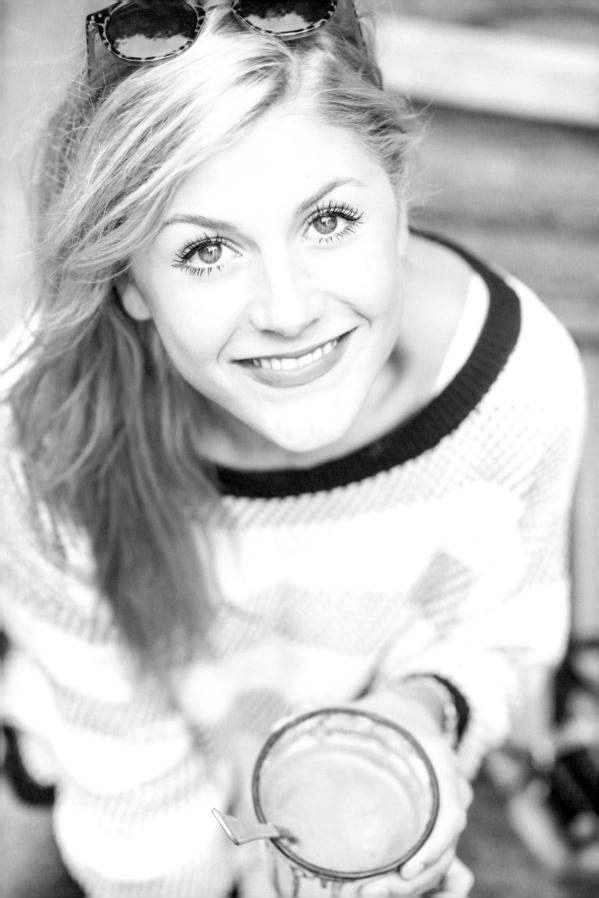

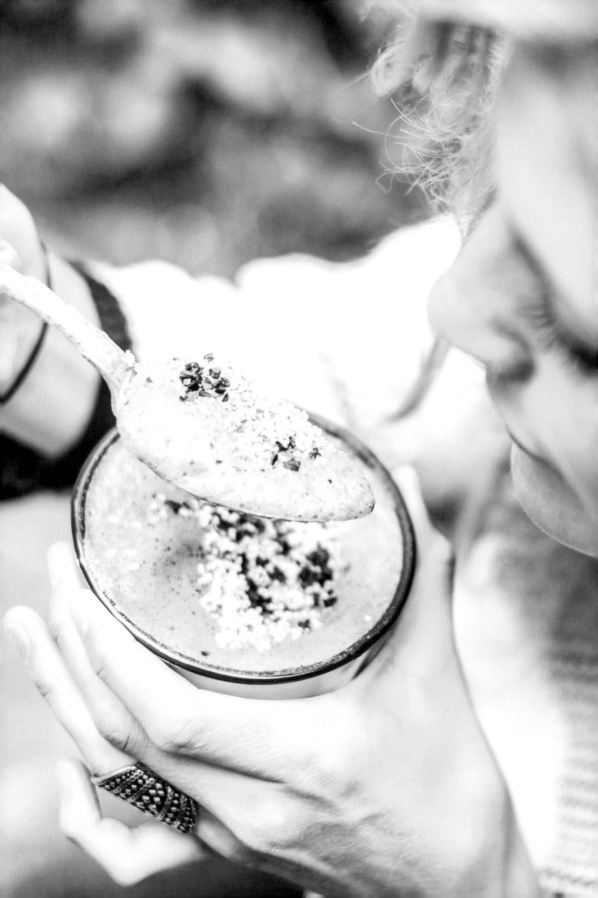

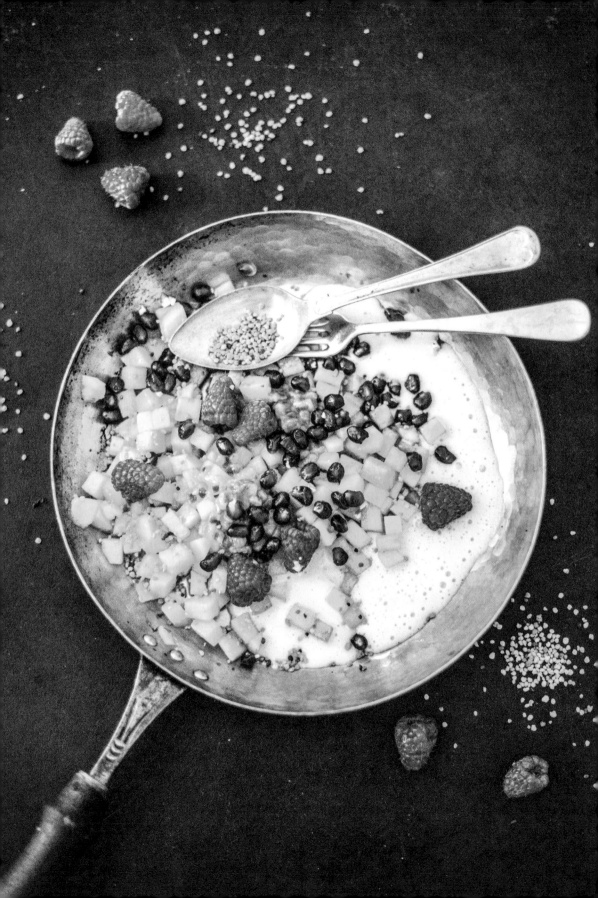

Sunny Fruit Salad on a Lemony Almond Foam

A fruit salad with that certain something.

Creating fruit salads is like experimenting with fashion. You should dare to try out new things, even if at first you might think that they don't go together at all. But you only know once you try it. This fruit salad is pretty tasty alone, but I felt that something was missing. This foam, which balances so well with the fruit used in the salad, was the finishing touch. When it comes to choosing fruit it's very important to use ripe fruit, since this is when the flavour, juiciness and natural sweetness really shine through.

SERVES 2-3 / GF, DF, VGN, RSF

FRUIT
1 ripe cantaloupe melon
1 ripe mango
2 passion fruits
seeds of ½ pomegranate
250 g (9 oz/2 cups) raspberries

FOAM
juice of 2 lemons
1½ tablespoons maple syrup or honey
1 tablespoon almond butter
pinch of salt

1 tablespoon bee pollen, to garnish

1   First, prepare the fruit. Peel the melon, cut it into quarters, remove the seeds, cut the flesh into dice and add into a bowl. Peel the mango, cut the flesh off the stone, dice and add to the bowl. Halve the passion fruits, scoop out the seeds and add to the bowl. Finally, add the pomegranate seeds and raspberries and carefully stir everything together.

2   To make the foam, pour the fresh lemon juice into a pan, add the maple syrup, almond butter and salt, and cook over a medium heat for 2–3 minutes. Mix with a hand blender or whisk to a light foam. The more you mix, the foamier it gets. Depending on how sour the lemons are you might have to add more maple syrup or a dash of milk.

3   Pour some of the foam into bowls, top with the fruit salad, garnish with bee pollen and serve.

TIP   If you want to serve the fruit salad cold, then cool it in the fridge for about 1 hour. Only prepare the foam right before serving. I really like the combination of the fresh fruit with the slightly warm foam!

Chocolate Truffles with Pistachio & Coconut Crunch

The best medicine for heart and soul.

If you have a weakness for chocolate and coconut, you will be excited to try out this recipe. The chocolate I make doesn't contain any sugar, preservatives or other unnatural ingredients. It's actually made with just three ingredients: raw cacao powder, coconut oil and coconut nectar. To add a little crunch, I add some home-made coconut chips and pistachios because I simply adore chocolate with some crunch. You're free to choose any topping you like though. If you prefer other kinds of nuts, add the ones you like. Dried fruit like berries, chopped dates or raisins are also great additions.

MAKES 8–10 TRUFFLES / GF, DF, VGN, RSF

CHOCOLATE

4 tablespoons coconut oil

4 tablespoons cacao powder

3–4 tablespoons coconut nectar

CRUNCH

3 tablespoons Sesame Coconut Chips (see page 96)

2 tablespoons soy or almond milk

pinch of salt

TOPPING IDEAS

almonds or hazelnuts, roasted

pistachios, crushed

1 To make the chocolate, melt the coconut oil over a medium heat in a small saucepan. Take off the heat, let the oil cool a bit, then add the cacao powder and coconut nectar and stir until well combined. The consistency should be similar to caramel. Taste with a spoon and, depending on how sweet you like it, add some more coconut nectar if necessary.

2 Add the crunch ingredients and stir well.

3 Spread the chocolate mixture onto some parchment paper into a square or rectangle 3–5 mm (¼ in) thick. Add your toppings of choice and put the chocolate into the freezer for at least 2 hours.

4 Once frozen, cut the chocolate into 6–8 equally sized strips and roll each strip into a ball with your hands. Sprinkle some crushed nuts on top or roll them into the balls as well.

5 Enjoy right away; the truffles soften very quickly. Otherwise, store them in the freezer (not the fridge) and take out 2–3 minutes before eating.

VARIATION   If you don't have coconut nectar to hand or can't find it at the health food store, sweeten with honey, agave, rice syrup or maple syrup. You will need to freeze the chocolate strips for a bit longer, as coconut nectar has a stickier and thicker consistency than the other sweeteners.

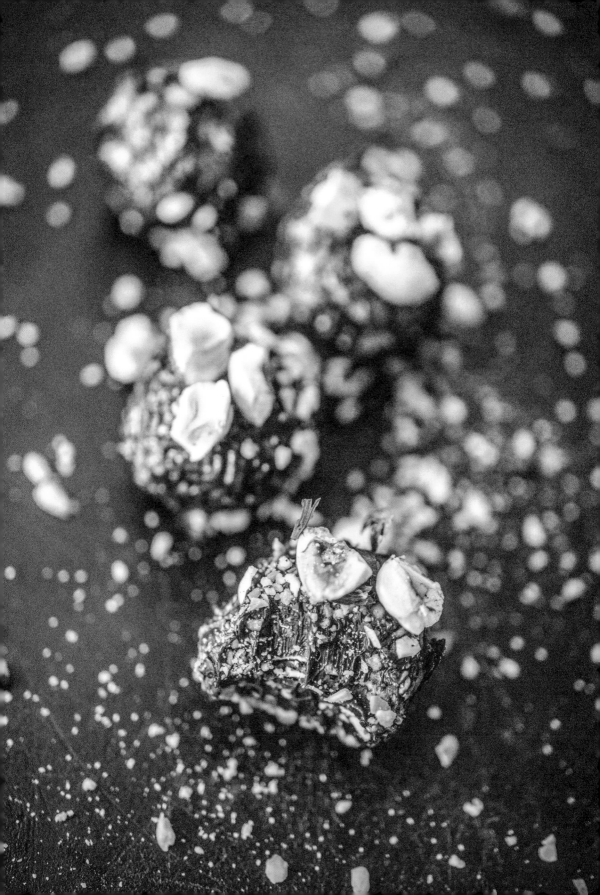

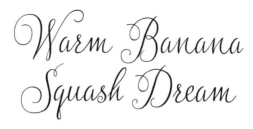

Warm Banana Squash Dream

Discovered in Thailand, reinvented in Switzerland.
When I was in Thailand, I went to a night food market in
Chiang Mai. It was full of delicious curries and traditional Thai dishes, but I wasn't too
keen on trying any of the desserts. However, I decided to give the cooked banana and
squash in coconut milk a try. And I think I had it almost every night after that as well.
Such a simple and delightful dessert, made with only a few nourishing and wholesome
ingredients. They also make the same dessert with banana and sweet potato, durian
or mango. I personally like the banana and squash combination the best.
Definitely worth a try!

SERVES 2 / GF, DF, VGN, RSF

BANANA & SQUASH

6–8 baby bananas or 2 large bananas

400 g (14 oz) butternut squash

250 ml (8½ fl oz) coconut water

250 ml (8½ fl oz) coconut milk

1 tablespoon almond or coconut butter

1–2 tablespoons coconut sugar,
   coconut nectar or rice syrup

pinch of salt

1 vanilla bean, seeds scraped

TOPPINGS

almonds, crushed

Sesame Coconut Chips (see page 96)

unsweetened cranberries

drizzle of coconut nectar (optional)

1   Peel the bananas and squash, and cut into 2–3 cm
(approx. 1 in) chunks.

2   In a large saucepan, bring the coconut water
and coconut milk to the boil. Add the banana and
butternut squash, reduce the heat, then add the remaining
ingredients. Cook over a medium heat for 15–20 minutes.
Stir carefully from time to time to avoid it burning at the
bottom of the pan.

3   If the mixture gets too thick, add another splash of
coconut water or coconut milk and turn down the heat a
bit. The banana and squash should soften to the point where
they almost melt in your mouth when you eat them.

4   Spoon the mixture into bowls, top with nuts, coconut
chips and cranberries, and drizzle a bit of coconut nectar
on top if desired. Serve and enjoy.

TIP   Don't forget to add the pinch of salt as it enhances the
sweetness as well as other flavours.

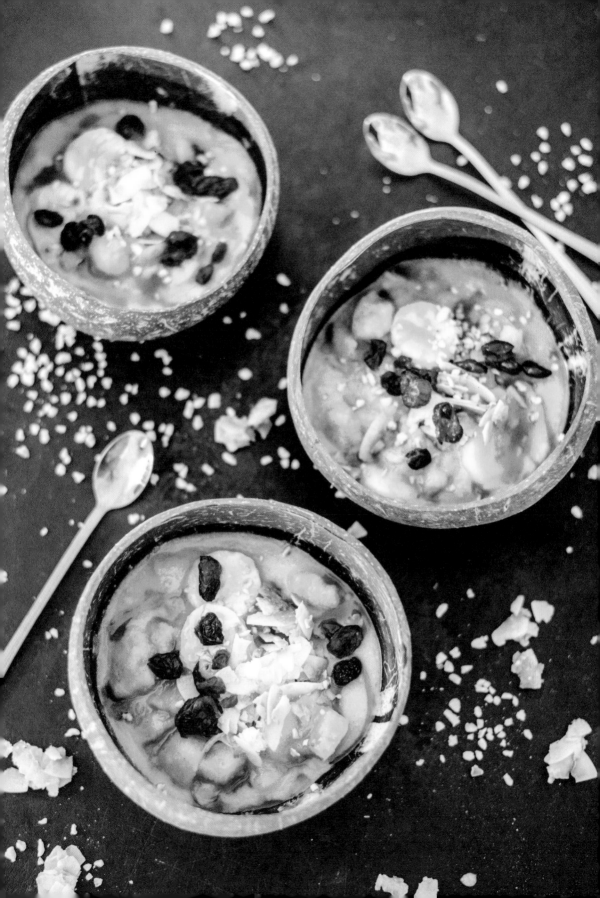

Banana Popsicle Runway

Made within minutes and eaten within seconds. Simply delicious!

It sometimes astonishes me how easy it is to create incredibly tasty and healthy treats with only a few ingredients, just like these popsicles. Of course, you could also run around the corner and buy an ice cream, but these popsicles are a must-must-try, especially for hot summer days. Adults love them just as much as kids. To make them in no time, make sure to always have some peeled and frozen banana halves in your freezer with popsicle sticks inserted. Then all you need to do is put on a chocolate coat, freshly designed by you, including the decoration.

──────────── MAKES 6-8 POPSICLES RSF*, (GF, DF, VGN)** ────────────

BANANAS

3–4 ripe bananas

wooden popsicle sticks

COATING

60–80 g (2–3 oz) min. 70% cocoa dark chocolate, or *dark chocolate sweetened with stevia

roasted and crushed nuts, e.g. hazelnuts, pistachios, cashews, almonds

dried berries, e.g. goji berries, mulberries, strawberries

Sesame Coconut Chips (see page 96)

1 teaspoon peanut butter (optional)

1   Peel the bananas, cut them in half, stick a wooden popsicle stick into each half and freeze for at least 2–3 hours.

2   Break the chocolate into pieces and melt it in a heatproof bowl over a saucepan of simmering water. Stir until smooth and take off the heat.

3   Add your toppings of choice onto small plates. Take the frozen banana halves out of the freezer, dip them in the dark chocolate, roll them in the toppings, then put them onto a plate with the sticks pointing up to set. The chocolate will harden very quickly because of the temperature difference.

4   For the peanut butter version, add a spoonful of the chocolate into a smaller bowl, stir in the peanut butter and dip the banana popsicle in it. Coat with nuts.

TIP   Roast the nuts before, which intensifies the nutty aroma and makes them crunchier! Roast in the oven for 10–15 minutes at 160°C (356°F/Gas 3), take them out, let them cool and then crush.

VARIATION   To make completely dairy-free, gluten-free, vegan popsicles, make the chocolate yourself. Melt 2 tablespoons of coconut oil, add 2 tablespoons of raw cacao powder and 2 tablespoons of maple syrup or sweetener of choice, stir well until smooth and keep warm on the stove over a low–medium heat. Dip the frozen banana in it.

**Depending on what chocolate you buy, you can get gluten-free, dairy-free and vegan chocolate. Simply check the ingredients.

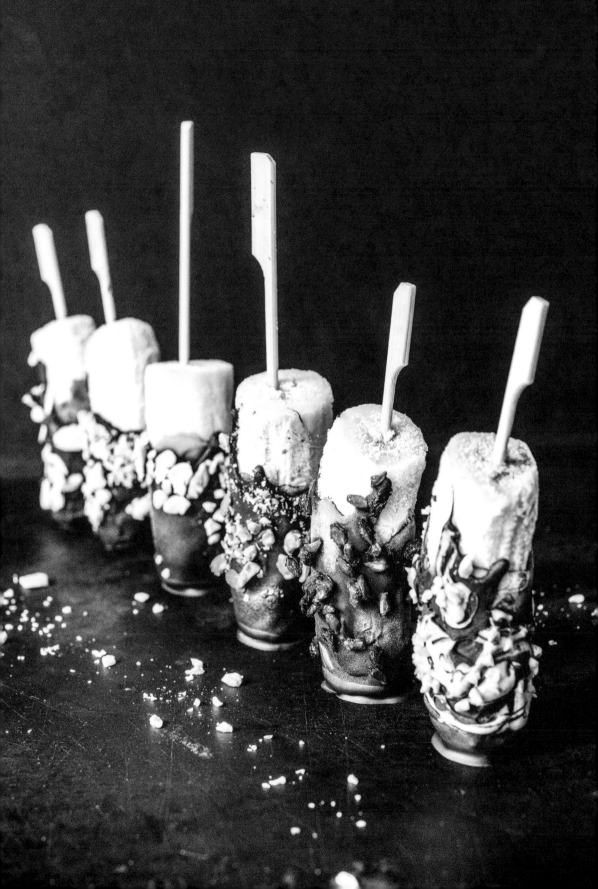

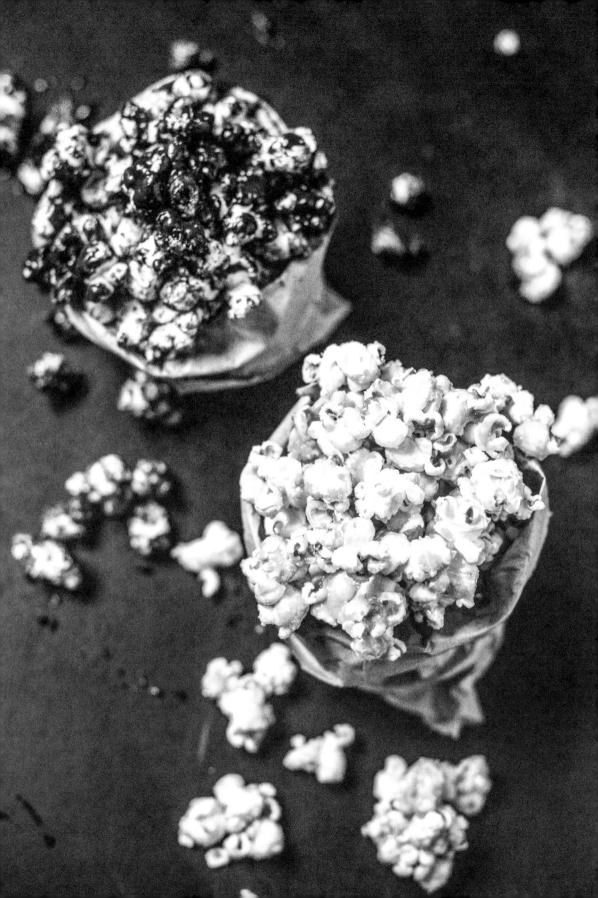

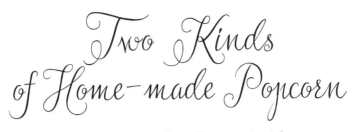

Two Kinds of Home-made Popcorn

Something to snack on for a movie night.

I have to admit, this popcorn might not look very healthy, but compared to the popcorn at the movies, drowning in butter or caramelised with sugar, it is.
My peanut and chocolate chia versions don't contain any refined sugar, butter or oil.
Another option to turn popcorn into a healthy snack is to pop it into the oven without any added oil. From now on, popcorn is no longer an unhealthy snack –
it's time to enjoy it again completely guilt-free!

SERVES 3-4 / GF, DF, RSF*

PEANUT POPCORN

3–4 tablespoons popping corn

1 tablespoon honey or rice syrup

1 tablespoon peanut butter

few drops of vanilla extract

CHOCOLATE CHIA POPCORN

3–4 tablespoons popping corn

50–70 g (2–2½ oz) min. 75% cocoa dark chocolate or *dark chocolate sweetened with stevia

1 tablespoon chia seeds

1 teaspoon maple syrup or sweetener of choice

few drops of vanilla extract

PEANUT POPCORN

Pop the popcorn in a popcorn machine, then transfer into a large mixing bowl. Put the honey or rice syrup, peanut butter and vanilla extract into a saucepan and melt together over a medium heat, stirring constantly. Pour the peanut mixture over the popcorn and with two spoons mix until well combined. Let it cool before serving.

CHOCOLATE CHIA POPCORN

Pop the popcorn in a popcorn machine, then transfer into a large mixing bowl. Break the chocolate into small pieces and melt it in a heatproof bowl over a saucepan of simmering water. Add the chia seeds, honey and vanilla extract, and stir until well combined. Pour the chocolate chia mixture over the popcorn, and with two spoons, mix until well combined. Let it cool before serving.

VARIATION   If you don't have a popcorn machine you can buy plain popcorn. Make sure to get a kind without salt or preservatives, and with no added oil (or as little as possible). The organic kinds are usually a good choice. The easiest, best and healthiest way to make popcorn is to make it with a popcorn machine where you don't have to add any oil at all and freshly popped corn is ready within a few minutes.

Watermelon Pizza Topped with Cashew Cream

Creativity knows no bounds.

This summer, I ate a whole small watermelon almost every day and didn't need anything else to eat for a few hours. One day, I felt like trying out something new, though, instead of simply cutting the watermelon in half and spooning it out. I started off by slicing the watermelon and then the idea of pizza immediately came to my mind. But what do I top it with? Maybe a cream and more fruit? Exactly! Yoghurt is always great to have with watermelon! To add some healthy fats and more creaminess, I also mixed cashews into the yoghurt that I spread on to the watermelon slice. Topping it with fresh berries and some pistachios not only adds some more juiciness and crunchiness, but also surprises friends and family with the look! Make sure to cool the watermelon slices in the fridge before making the pizzas.

SERVES 1–2 / GF, DF*, VGN*, RSF

WATERMELON & TOPPINGS

2–3 round slices of watermelon, 2 cm (¾ in) thick

fruit and berries of choice

pistachios, crushed

CASHEW CREAM

50 g (2 oz) cashews

2–3 teaspoons maple syrup or sweetener of choice

3 tablespoons Greek yoghurt or *soy yoghurt

1–2 teaspoons nut butter, e.g. pistachio butter (see page 36)

few drops of vanilla extract

1   Put all the ingredients for the cashew cream into a food processor and blend for 2–3 minutes until smooth and creamy.

2   Spread the cashew cream evenly on to the slices of watermelon and top with your chosen fruit and berries, and the pistachios. Cut into slices and serve.

TIP   Summer berries make a delicious topping. Also, this is a great idea for a children's birthday party. The kids love it and they can all make their own watermelon pizza creations. Plus, it's healthy!

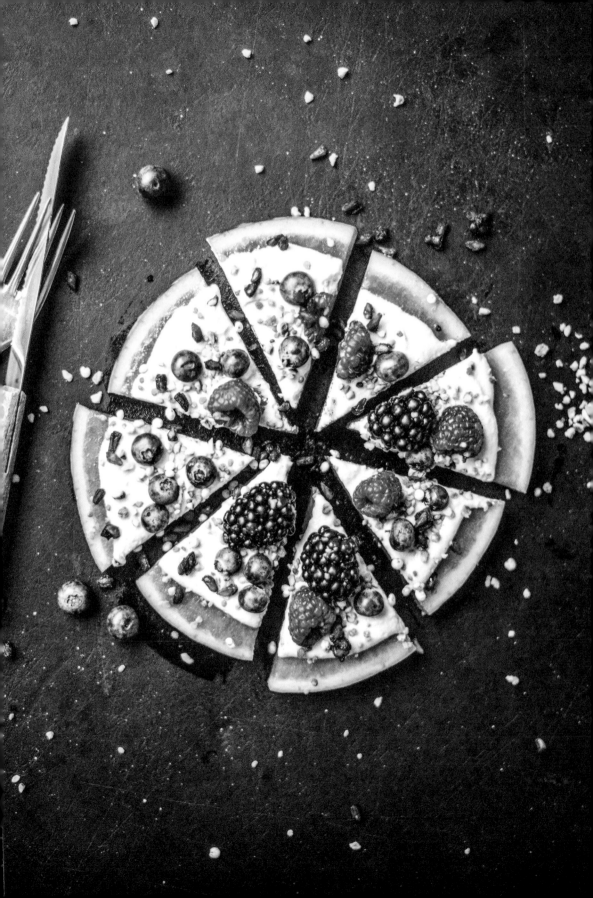

Superfood Cacao Energy Balls

Small, but full of power and taste!

No matter how balanced and healthy your diet is, if you are always snacking between meals with muesli, chocolate bars, crisps (chips), crackers or other unhealthy and processed foods, it leads you nowhere. But what can you eat as a snack if you're on the go or working out that is actually healthy and will satisfy your hunger and cravings? These superfood balls are just perfect.

—————————— MAKES 16-20 ENERGY BALLS / GF, DF, VGN, RSF ——————————

CACAO BALLS

50 g (2 oz) almonds

50 g (2 oz) cashews

50 g (2 oz) oats (oatmeal) (gluten-free)

20 g (¾ oz) sunflower seeds

20 g (¾ oz) pumpkin seeds

2 tablespoons shredded coconut

1 tablespoon linseeds

50 g (2 oz) unsweetened chocolate or vanilla
protein powder

4 Medjool dates, pitted

1 tablespoon maple syrup or sweetener
of choice

1 tablespoon peanut or almond butter

2 tablespoons raw cacao powder

few drops of vanilla extract

TOPPING IDEAS

pumpkin seeds

sunflower seeds

raw cacao powder

goji berries

roasted flaked (slivered) almonds

chia seeds

shredded coconut

puffed amaranth

1   Preheat the oven to 180°C (350°F/Gas 4).

2   Line a baking tray with parchment paper and spread the almonds, cashews, oats, sunflower seeds and pumpkin seeds on top. Roast for about 15–20 minutes, take out of the oven and let them cool.

3   Put the roasted nuts, oats and seeds into a blender or food processor along with the remaining ingredients and blend well into a doughy, thick mixture. If the mixture is too dry, add another Medjool date or a small dash of water.

4   Scrape the doughy mixture out of the blender or food processor and form it into one large ball. Flatten the ball with your hands a little and cut it into 16–20 equally sized pieces. Form the pieces into balls with your hands and, if you want, roll them in whatever toppings you prefer. My favourite topping is definitely chia seeds!

5   Store in the fridge. They're best when eaten slightly chilled but you can also take them out and about with you.

VARIATION   Feel free to use whichever type of protein powder you like. I personally love organic chocolate protein powder but you could also use soy, whey, hemp protein, pea protein … whichever you prefer!

STORAGE   You can store the superfood balls in the fridge in an airtight jar for about 1 week. Or you could double the quantities and freeze half of the balls so that you always have a nourishing snack ready to grab. Take them out of the freezer and thaw for about 5 minutes before eating.

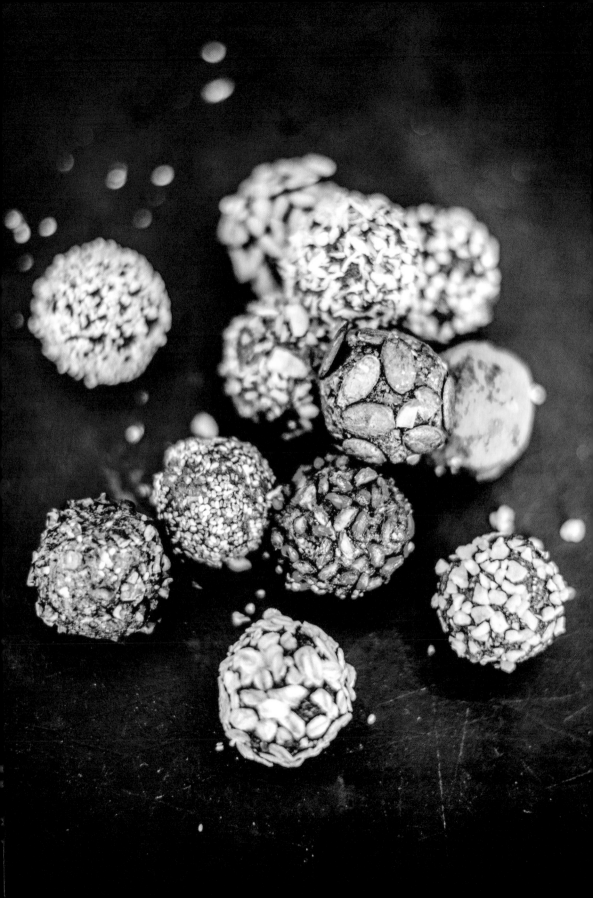

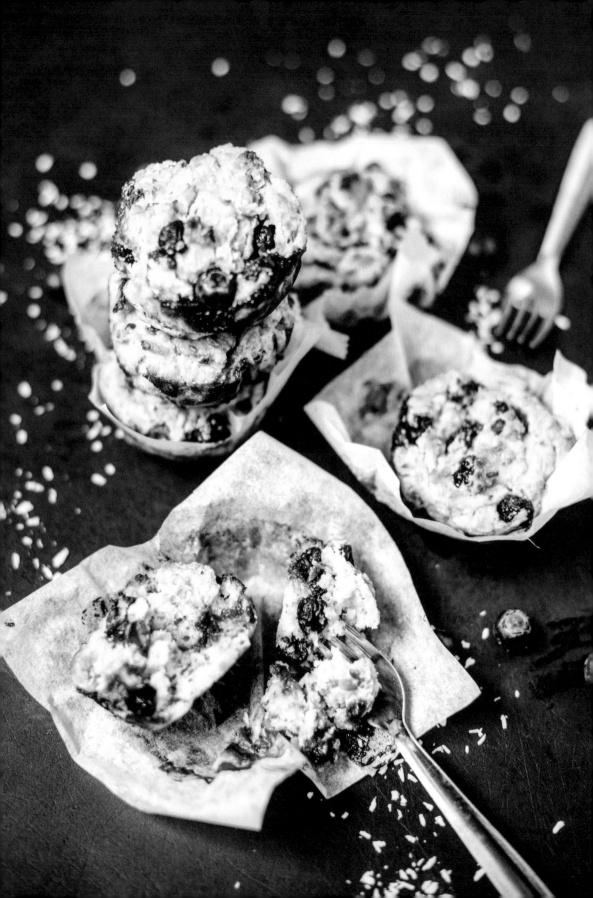

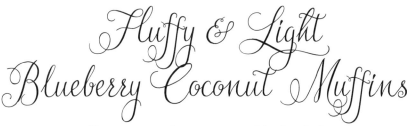

Fluffy & Light Blueberry Coconut Muffins

You can never have too many blueberries!

A muffin is something we all love to have from time to time, preferably with a good cup of coffee or tea. But they usually contain a lot of sugar, white flour and other ingredients it is best to stay away from. When you make muffins yourself, you know exactly what is in them and you can also replace the unhealthy ingredients with healthier alternatives. I replace the white flour with amaranth flour and coconut flour, both of which are gluten-free. The yoghurt keeps the muffins moist, and the combination of blueberries and coconut transports you to paradise.

———————— MAKES 8 MUFFINS / GF, (DF, VGN*), RSF ————————

1 ripe banana

180 g (6 oz) Greek or *soy yoghurt

1–2 tablespoons maple syrup

1 tablespoon almond butter

1 teaspoon vanilla extract

1 tablespoon coconut oil, melted

8–10 tablespoons oats (oatmeal) (gluten-free)

2 tablespoons shredded coconut

2 tablespoons amaranth flour

1 tablespoon coconut flour

2 teaspoons gluten-free baking powder

pinch of salt

150 g (5 oz) fresh or frozen blueberries

Greek yoghurt, to serve

drizzle of maple syrup or honey, to serve

blueberries, to serve

1　Preheat the oven to 180°C (350°F/Gas 4). Line a muffin tin with 8 muffin cases.

2　In a bowl, mash the banana to a purée with a fork. Add the yoghurt, maple syrup, almond butter, vanilla extract and melted coconut oil. Stir well.

3　Grind the oats into a flour using a food precessor. Tip the oat flour into a separate large mixing bowl then mix in the remaining ingredients except for the blueberries. Pour the wet mixture into the dry mixture and stir until just combined – don't over-mix. Briefly stir in the blueberries.

4　Fill the muffin cases equally with the batter and bake in the lower part of the oven for 25–35 minutes until golden brown.

5　Take the muffins out of the oven. Let them cool slightly and eat while still warm, or leave to cool completely. Take a muffin with you as a snack or serve it with a spoonful of Greek yoghurt, a drizzle of maple syrup or honey and fresh blueberries.

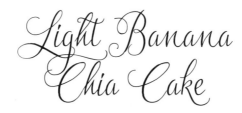

Light Banana Chia Cake

For breakfast, as a snack or for dessert: always a hit!

Nutty but still so moist: this banana chia cake is one of my favourite recipes. It's perfect for a quick breakfast with some home-made peanut butter, after a good workout to fuel up or simply for dessert served with some fresh banana ice cream. Whenever I have guests over, this cake is always a winner. And the good thing about it is that everyone can eat it because it's completely gluten-free, dairy-free, vegan and doesn't contain any refined sugar. It's super tasty to eat fresh out of the oven when it's still a bit warm. The most delicious banana cake you'll ever have.

MAKES 1 CAKE (APPROX. 8-10 PIECES) / GF, DF, VGN, RSF

BANANA CHIA CAKE

2–3 ripe bananas

4 tablespoons chia seeds

150 ml (5 fl oz) milk of choice, e.g. soy, almond, rice milk

2–3 teaspoons maple syrup or sweetener of choice

1 vanilla bean, seeds scraped

1 tablespoon coconut oil

1 tablespoon peanut butter or nut butter of choice

4 tablespoons ground almonds

4 tablespoons amaranth flour or other gluten-free flour, e.g. quinoa or millet

1 teaspoon gluten-free baking powder

1 tablespoon coconut flour

pinch of salt

50 g (2 oz) whole almonds or walnuts

TOPPINGS

1 banana

crushed nuts of choice

drizzle of honey or maple syrup

1   For the cake, peel the bananas, cut them into slices and put them into a large bowl. Mash them with a fork to a purée. Add the chia seeds, milk maple syrup, vanilla, coconut oil and peanut butter, and stir until well combined. Let the mixture stand for about 1 hour so that the chia seeds can soak up the liquid and swell.

2   Preheat the oven to 180°C (350°F/Gas 4) and line a 900 g (2 lb) loaf tin with parchment paper.

3   In another large bowl, mix together all the other ingredients and add to the banana mixture. Stir gently until just combined. Don't over-mix.

4   Pour the mixture into the prepared loaf tin. Peel the banana for the topping and slice diagonally. Lay on top of the cake, sprinkle over crushed nuts, and drizzle some honey on top. Bake in the lower part of the oven for 35–40 minutes.

5   Turn off the oven, open the oven door a bit and let the cake cool or serve slightly warm.

VARIATION   If you don't have coconut flour at home, simply add another tablespoon of ground almonds to the cake mixture. To add a little colour and more fruitiness, add 150–200 g (5–7 oz) of berries to the mixture.

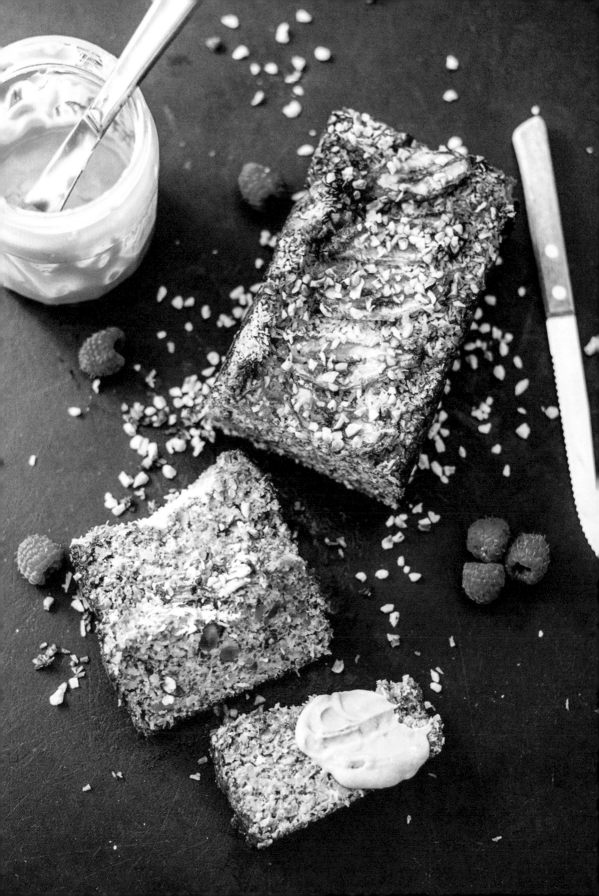

Raw Bars with an Almond Base to Die For

My signature dessert!

These delicious, sweet, ice-cold but oh-so-creamy bars quickly become a favourite for everyone after tasting them. I love having a batch in the freezer ready to offer to my visitors. You only need to thaw them for a few minutes until they reach the consistency that will melt in your mouth and make you think that you're eating cake and ice cream at the same time. Can it get any better? Pay attention though: they're very addictive! One piece quickly becomes two or three. But you know what? I don't care and you shouldn't care either — these bars are too good to only have one.

MAKES APPROX. 18 PIECES / GF, DF*, VGN*, RSF**

ALMOND BASE

200 g (7 oz) almonds

1 tablespoon coconut oil

1 tablespoon peanut or almond butter

1½ tablespoons maple syrup or sweetener of choice

pinch of salt

1 tablespoon shredded coconut

few drops of vanilla extract

CREAM

2 ripe bananas

1 tablespoon maple syrup or sweetener of choice

200 g (7 oz) low-fat quark or *soy yoghurt/quark

2 tablespoons peanut butter

2 teaspoons almond butter

2 teaspoons coconut oil

few drops of vanilla extract

TOPPING

50 g (2 oz) min. 75% cocoa dark chocolate or **dark chocolate sweetened with stevia

2 teaspoons coconut oil

fresh blueberries or berries of choice

crushed almonds or cashews

cacao nibs

1   For the almond base, put all the ingredients into a blender or food processor and blend to a coarse mixture that sticks together. A strong blender or processor is required.

2   Line a 20 × 20 cm (8 × 8 in) square baking tray with parchment paper. Spoon in the almond mixture and press down with your hands to an even thickness.

3   For the cream, peel the bananas, cut them into small pieces and mix into a smooth and creamy mixture with the remaining ingredients. Pour onto the almond base and smooth out. Freeze for 2 hours.

4   After 2 hours, break the chocolate for the topping into small pieces and melt in a small saucepan together with the coconut oil over a low heat. Turn off the heat and keep warm on the stove.

5   Take the tray out of the freezer, cut the dessert into 15–18 equally sized pieces and drizzle the hot chocolate on top. The chocolate will set immediately on the frozen bars. Garnish with berries, crushed nuts and cacao nibs.

TIP   Put the bars back into the freezer and only leave out as many as you want to eat right away. The bars soften and melt very quickly if you leave them out for too long. Before serving, take them out of the freezer and thaw for 2–5 minutes so that the cream softens a bit.

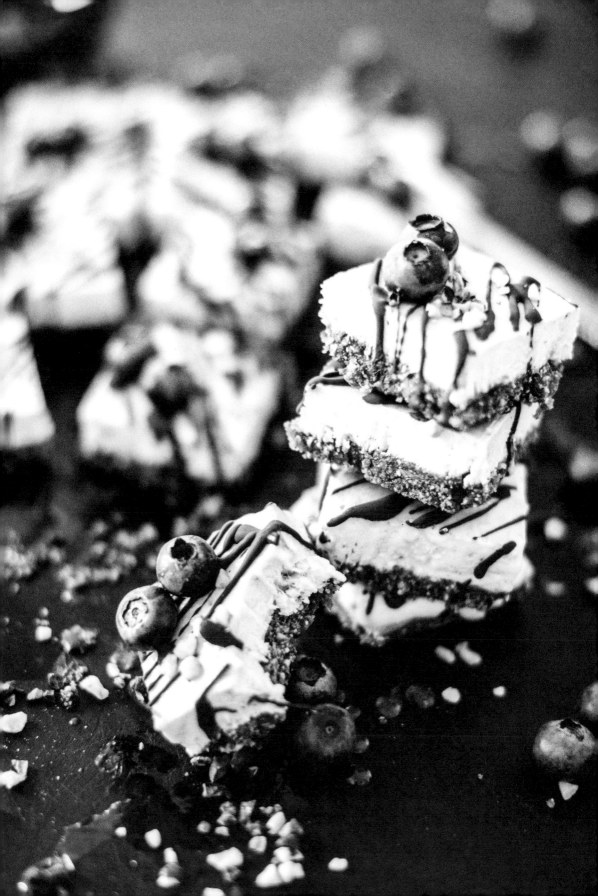

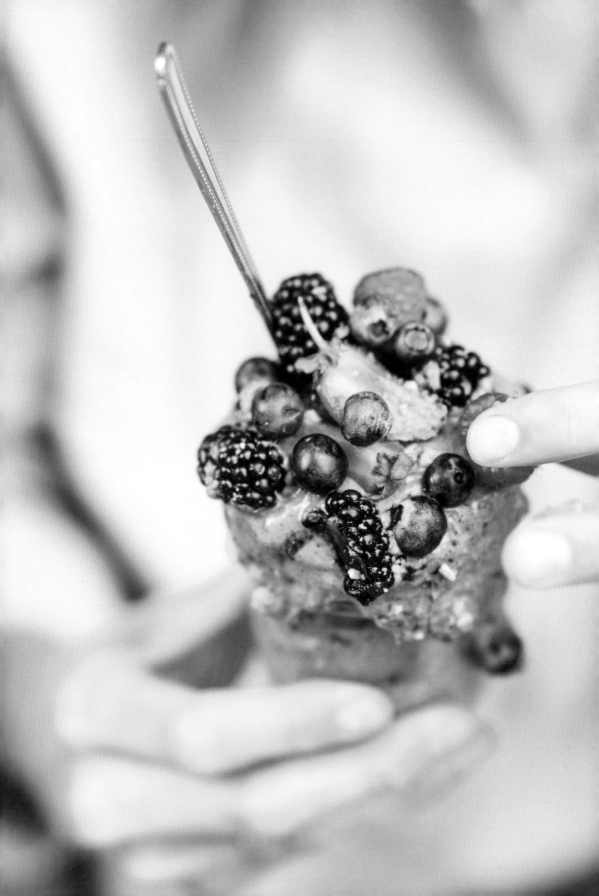

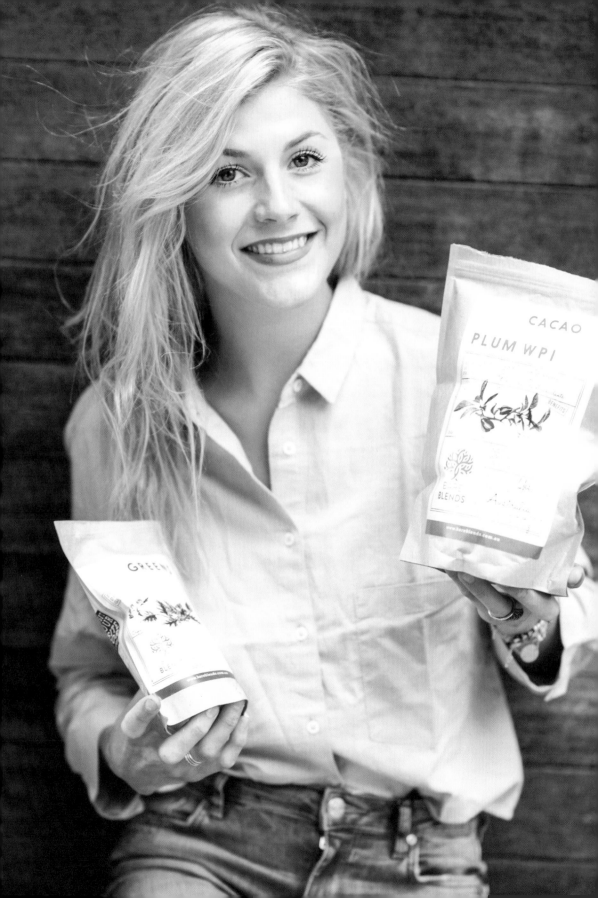

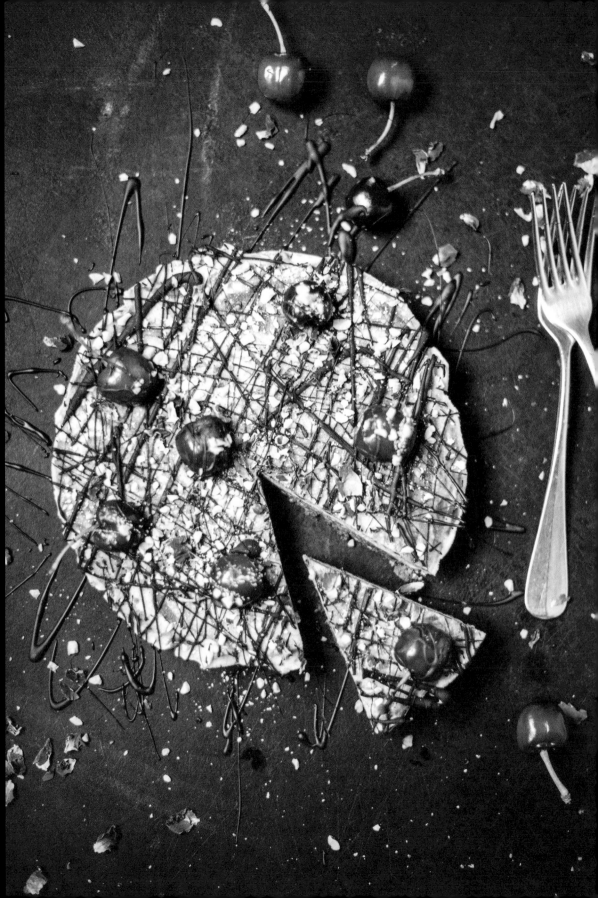

Ice-Cold Banana, Cherry & Chocolate Cake

... and a topping that transforms it into a real work of art.

I've always been a fan of raw cakes, especially the frozen ones. It's a nice mix of both having a piece of cake and ice cream without overindulging at all. Another benefit is that you can keep the cake in the freezer and cut off individually sized pieces whenever you feel like it. The base is made of nuts and dates, and the cream on top is a mix of bananas and yoghurt. No sugar added, no flour, no butter, no cream.

—————— MAKES 1 CAKE (APPROX. 20 CM/ 8 IN) / GF, DF*, VGN*, RSF** ——————

BASE

14 dates, pitted

200 ml (7 fl oz) water

6 tablespoons ground almonds

3 tablespoons cashews

3 tablespoons raw cacao powder

1½ tablespoons maple syrup or sweetener
  of choice

CREAM

2 ripe bananas

2 tablespoons shredded coconut

1 tablespoon almond butter

2 tablespoons cashews

4–5 tablespoons low-fat yoghurt or
  *soy yoghurt

1 tablespoon maple syrup or sweetener
  of choice

CHERRY-CREAM

10 cherries, pitted

3 tablespoons low-fat yoghurt or *soy yoghurt

2 tablespoons maple syrup or sweetener
  of choice

TOPPINGS

20 g (¾ oz) min. 75% cocoa dark chocolate
  or **dark chocolate sweetened with stevia

2 teaspoons coconut oil

cherries

crushed nuts of choice

dried rose petals

1   To make the base, bring 60–80 ml (2–2½ fl oz) water to the boil, take it off the heat, add the dates and soak them for 5–10 minutes. Drain and transfer them to a powerful blender or food processor with the remaining ingredients and blend to a coarse mixture that sticks together. You should be able to easily form the mixture into a ball. If the dough is too dry or doesn't stick together, add a splash of water; if the dough is too wet, add another spoonful of ground almonds.

2   Line a 20 cm (8 in) round cake tin with baking parchment. Pour the mixture into the centre of the tin and press down evenly right to the edges of the cake tin.

3   For the cream, peel and slice the bananas, and put them into a blender. Add the remaining ingredients and blend for 4–5 minutes until smooth and creamy. Pour onto the base and smooth out.

4   For the cherry cream, purée the cherries, yoghurt and maple syrup until smooth. Drizzle the cream on top of the banana mixture in circles. With a fork, stir through the mixture a few times to make a swirl. Freeze the cake for about 1 hour.

5   For the topping, melt the chocolate and coconut oil in a heatproof bowl over a saucepan of hot water. Take the cake out of the freezer, add the cherries on top and, with a spoon, drizzle the chocolate in a criss-cross pattern over the whole cake. Sprinkle over the nuts. Freeze for at least another hour.

6   Take the cake out of the freezer about 10 minutes before serving. Scatter with rose petals, cut into slices, close your eyes and enjoy!

Pancakes with Carob & Vanilla Cream

You can't say no to pancakes!

If it were up to me, pancakes would officially be on the menu of every Sunday breakfast or brunch meet-up. There's nothing like sitting at the table with family and friends with a selection of pancakes and toppings on the table. All natural, fresh and home-made ingredients of course, and, just like this recipe, free of refined sugar, white flour and butter. Using only quinoa and amaranth flour makes these pancakes gluten-free as well. You can never go wrong with these pancakes; they will quickly put a smile on anyone's face and they're perfect to share.

SERVES 2 (MAKES 8-10 PANCAKES) / GF, DF *, VGN*, RSF

PANCAKES

70 g (2½ oz) quinoa flakes or flour

2 tablespoons amaranth flour

2 teaspoons gluten-free baking powder

pinch of salt

2 teaspoons instant coffee powder

1–1½ tablespoons raw cacao powder

1 banana, ripe

2 teaspoons coconut oil, plus extra for frying

1 tablespoon maple syrup or sweetener of choice

2 egg whites

250 ml (8½ fl oz) milk of choice, e.g. soy, almond, rice milk

coconut oil, for frying

CAROB CREAM

250 g low-fat Greek yoghurt or *soy yoghurt

1 tablespoon maple syrup or sweetener of choice

1 tablespoon carob powder

1 vanilla bean, seeds scraped

TOPPINGS

1 tablespoon puffed quinoa

1 tablespoon cacao nibs

2 fresh figs, sliced

berries of choice

1   For the pancakes, add the quinoa flakes or flour into a bowl along with the amaranth flour, baking powder, salt, instant coffee powder and raw cacao powder, and stir until well combined. Peel and slice the banana into another bowl, mash it with a fork and add the remaining ingredients. Stir until well combined. Add the wet mixture to the dry mixture and stir to a thickish batter that easily falls off the spoon. If that's not the case, add another splash of milk and stir again. Let it stand for at least 10 minutes.

2   For the carob cream, put all the ingredients into a bowl, stir until well combined and cool in the fridge.

3   In a large frying pan (skillet), heat up some coconut oil on a a medium heat. To make pancakes 10–12 cm (4–5 in) in diameter, drop 1 tablespoon of batter for each pancake into the pan and fry for 1–2 minutes until golden brown and bubbles form. Flip and fry on the other side until golden brown. Transfer to a plate.

4   Either serve the pancakes separately with the carob cream and toppings or make a pancake stack by spreading a spoon of carob cream on to every pancake and layering them up. Garnish with puffed quinoa, cacao nibs, figs and fresh fruit.

VARIATION   If you can't find quinoa flakes or flour, either just use amaranth flour or replace it with millet flour, ground oats or wholemeal spelt flour (not gluten-free).

NOTE   You will find carob powder at health food stores.

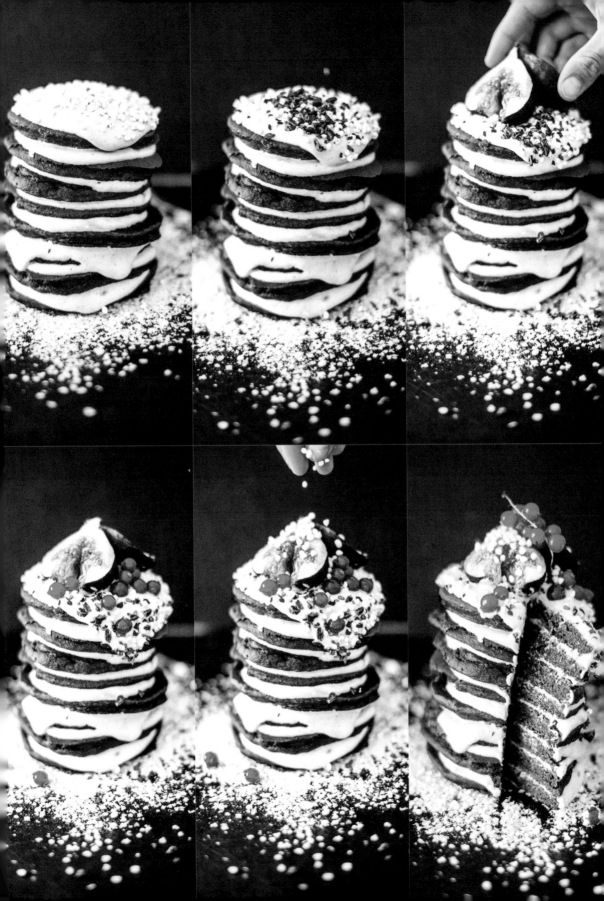

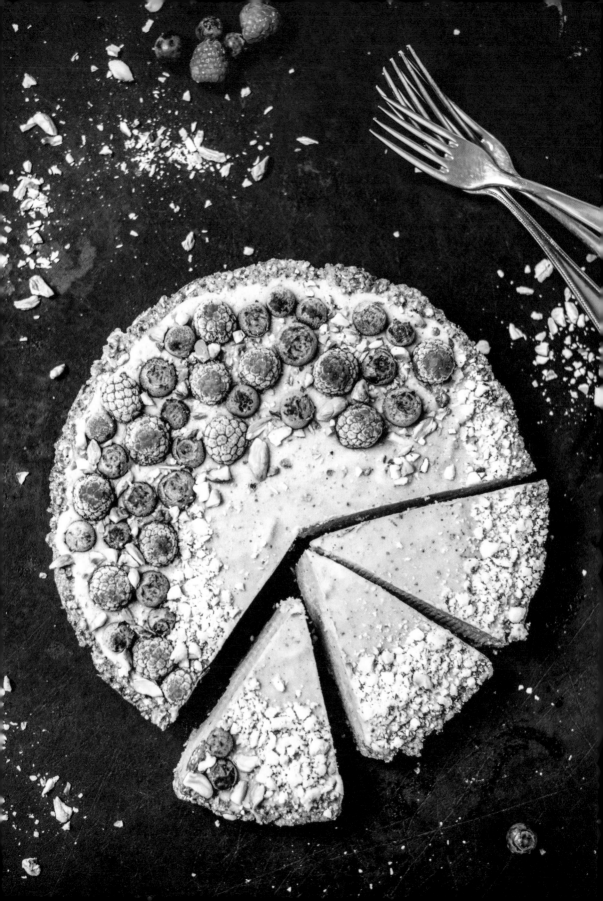

Raw Lime & Pistachio Cake with Cashew & Date Base

Nutty and refreshing at the same time!

I always like to make my raw cakes gluten-, dairy- and refined-sugar-free. This way there is something for everybody. This is a cake for every season: in summer you can garnish it with berries and in winter with roasted nuts and dried cranberries. The cake itself is really nutty and therefore also pretty high in calories, but nuts contain healthy fats, which our bodies need. Of all the nuts, pistachios and cashews are the lowest in calories. Their flavour comes out a lot better if you roast them beforehand.

―――――― MAKES 1 CAKE (APPROX. 25 CM/10 IN) / GF, *DF, *VGN, RSF ――――――

BASE

6 Medjool dates or 12 small dates, pitted

200 g (7 oz) cashews

2–3 teaspoons almond butter

40–60 ml (1½–2 fl oz) water

1 tablespoon maple syrup or sweetener of choice

few drops of vanilla extract

CREAM

350 g (12 oz) *soy yoghurt or natural yoghurt

100 g (3½ oz) pistachios

2 ripe bananas, peeled

1 tablespoon almond butter

1½ tablespoons coconut oil

3 tablespoons maple syrup or sweetener of choice

zest and juice of 2 limes

few drops of vanilla extract

pinch of salt

TOPPINGS

fresh or frozen berries

pistachios, roasted and crushed

cashews, roasted and crushed

1   To make the base, bring some water to the boil, pour it into a bowl and soak the dates for 5–10 minutes (the longer, the better).

2   Put the cashews into a powerful blender or food processor and grind. Drain the soaked dates and add them to the cashews along with the rest of the ingredients. Blend to a coarse dough. Add a splash of water if the mixture is too thick; add more ground cashews if the mixture is too moist.

3   Line a 25 cm (10 in) round cake tin with parchment paper. Add the base mixture and evenly press down with your hands so that the mixture reaches about 1.5 cm (½ in) up the side of the tin.

4   For the cream, add all the ingredients into a food processor and blend for at least 5–6 minutes until smooth and creamy. Pour on top of the base and smooth out with a spatula. Put into the freezer for at least 1 hour before you add the toppings. This way the toppings will stay on top of the slightly frozen cream and not sink into it.

5   Take the cake out of the freezer, garnish with berries and crushed nuts and freeze for another 2 hours.

6   Remove the cake from the freezer, thaw for about 10 minutes and cut into slices. Put any slices that you don't want to serve straight back into the freezer.

TIP   The best way to store the cake is to cut it into slices and store them in the freezer. Then you don't have to thaw the whole cake every time you want a piece. Before you eat a slice, make sure to thaw it for 10–15 minutes. You should easily be able to stick a fork in it. If you want the cake to be creamier, thaw for about 20–35 minutes.

Nutty Sweet Potato & Buckwheat Brownies

Brownies like you've never had them before.

Brownies – who doesn't love them? Of course, sometimes we just need to treat ourselves to a real brownie made with butter, more butter, chocolate and sugar. But when you have the option to make brownies with healthy and nutritious ingredients, you can make and enjoy them more often without over-indulging. In this recipe, the sweet potato gives the moist texture, holds everything together and adds some natural sweetness.

MAKES APPROX 18 BROWNIES / GF, DF, VGN, RSF

BROWNIES

1 large sweet potato

8 Medjool dates, pitted

2 ripe bananas

few drops of vanilla extract

2–3 tablespoons sweetener of choice
(preferably maple or rice syrup)

2 tablespoons peanut or almond butter

1 tablespoon coconut oil

splash of milk of choice, e.g. soy, almond, rice
milk (optional)

4 tablespoons ground almonds

100 g (3½ oz) whole almonds or walnuts

6 tablespoons raw cacao powder or
4 tablespoons raw cacao powder with
2 tablespoons carob powder

4 tablespoons buckwheat seeds

2 teaspoons gluten-free baking powder

pinch of salt

TOPPINGS

2 tablespoons buckwheat seeds

2 tablespoons crushed nuts of choice

drizzle of maple syrup or sweetener of choice

Healthy Chocolate Mousse (see page 208)
(optional)

fresh berries of choice (optional)

1   Preheat the oven to 190 °C (375°F/Gas 5) and line a 25 × 25 cm (10 × 10 in) square baking tin with parchment paper.

2   To make the brownies, bring a medium-sized saucepan of water to the boil. Peel and dice the sweet potato, and add to the boiling water together with the dates. Cook for 10–15 minutes until soft.

3   Put the bananas, vanilla, maple or rice syrup, nut butter and coconut oil into a food processor and blend until smooth. Drain the sweet potato and dates and add them to the banana mixture. Blend again until creamy. If the mixture is too thick, add a splash of milk. Pour into a bowl.

4   Add the remaining brownie ingredients to another bowl and stir well. Add the dry mixture to the wet mixture and carefully stir until well combined.

5   Transfer the dough into the prepared tin and smooth out evenly with a spatula. Top with the buckwheat seeds and crushed nuts and drizzle some maple syrup over the batter.

6   Bake for 30–35 minutes. The surface should be slightly browned and crispy when you touch it. Take out of the oven and let it cool. Cut into squares and either serve when they're still a little bit warm or let them cool completely. Spread some chocolate mousse over the brownies and top with berries to serve, if you like.

STORE   You can store the brownies in an airtight container in the fridge for up to 4–5 days. They're a perfect snack if you feel like eating cake and want to satisfy your sweet tooth. You can also wrap them in cling film (plastic wrap) and individually store them in the fridge to take away.

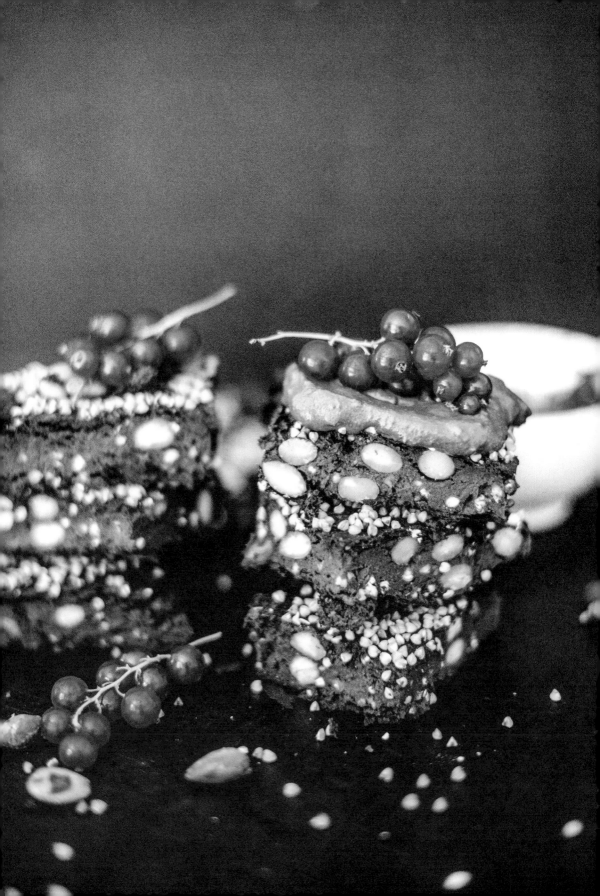

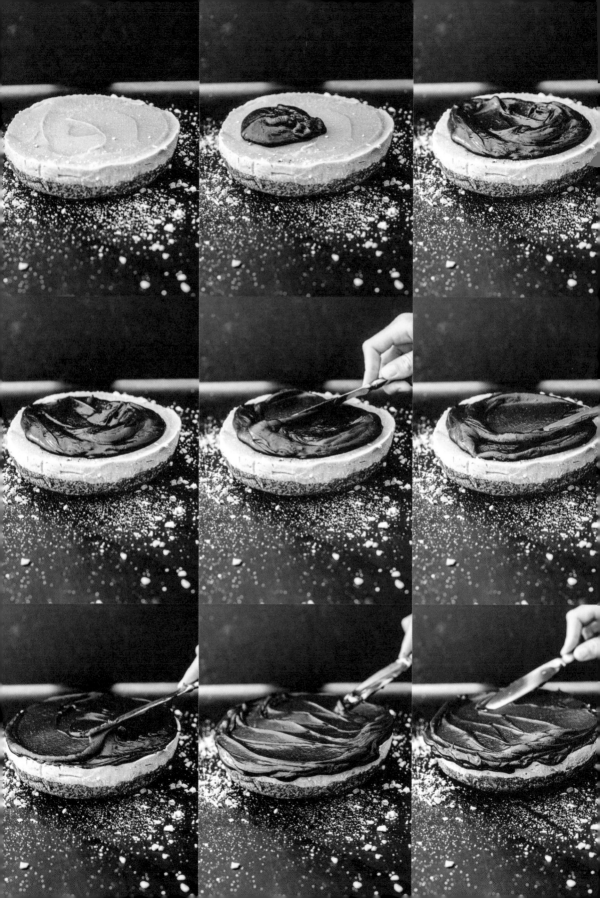

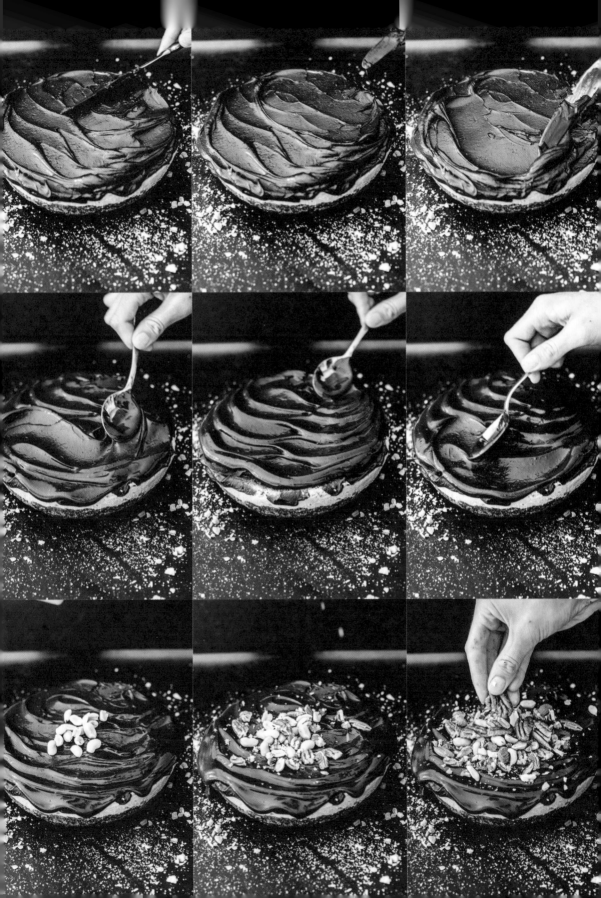

Divine Nougat Cheesecake Topped with Chocolate Sauce

A labour of love but worth every single minute of it!
My version of cheesecake simply had to be in this book and I feel like it's
the perfect recipe to end with. It shows how something we might think is unhealthy at
first glance can actually be both healthy and delicious.

MAKES 1 CAKE (APPROX. 26 CM/ 10 IN) / GF, DF, VGN, RSF

FILLING

150 g (5 oz) cashews, soaked
100 g (3½ oz) peanuts, soaked
250–300 ml (8½–10 fl oz) plant milk of
   choice, soy/almond or rice milk
pinch of salt
2 tablespoons coconut oil
2 tablespoons maple syrup or sweetener
   of choice
1 vanilla bean, seeds scraped

BASE

6 Medjool dates or 12 small dates, pitted
100 g (3½ oz) pecans
150 g (5 oz) ground almonds
2 tablespoons maple syrup or sweetener
   of choice
1 tablespoon coconut oil

CHOCOLATE

5 tablespoons coconut oil
6 tablespoons raw cacao powder
5 tablespoons rice syrup or sweetener
   of choice
pinch of salt
50–100 ml (2–2½ fl oz) soy, almond or
   rice milk

TOPPINGS

handful of nuts, roasted
1 tablespoon maple syrup

1   In a large bowl, soak the cashews and peanuts for the filling in water overnight or for at least 2–3 hours.

2   Line a 26 cm (10 in) round cake tin with parchment paper and preheat the oven to 160°C (320°F/Gas 3).

3   For the base, put the dates into a bowl, cover with boiling water and soak for at least 10 minutes. Roast the pecans in the oven for about 20 minutes. Take out of the oven and cool slightly. Transfer the nuts to a powerful blender or food processor and blend with the rest of the ingredients for the base into a slightly thick and sticky mixture. Spoon the mixture into the prepared cake tin and press down evenly with your hands. Put the base into the freezer.

4   For the filling, drain the soaked nuts and add to a food processor with the remaining ingredients. Blend to a smooth and creamy mixture for at least 6–8 minutes. Take the base out of the freezer, spoon the filling on top and smooth out evenly. Freeze for another 2 hours.

5   Once the cheesecake is frozen, start making the chocolate. Heat up the coconut oil over a medium heat until completely melted, take off the heat and add the raw cacao powder, sweetener and salt. Stir until it reaches the consistency of thick melted chocolate. For a more bitter chocolate taste, add 50–70 ml (2–2½ fl oz) of milk and stir again. If you prefer the taste of milkier chocolate, add 100 ml (3½ fl oz) of milk instead.

6   For the topping, put the nuts into a small saucepan together with the maple syrup and caramelise over a low–medium heat. Stir well, set aside and let it cool completely.

7   Take the cheesecake out of the freezer, spread the chocolate on top, garnish with the caramelised nuts and freeze for another 30 minutes. Remove from the freezer, rinse a knife with hot water and cut into slices. (If the cheesecake is still too hard, thaw for a few minutes and then slice.)

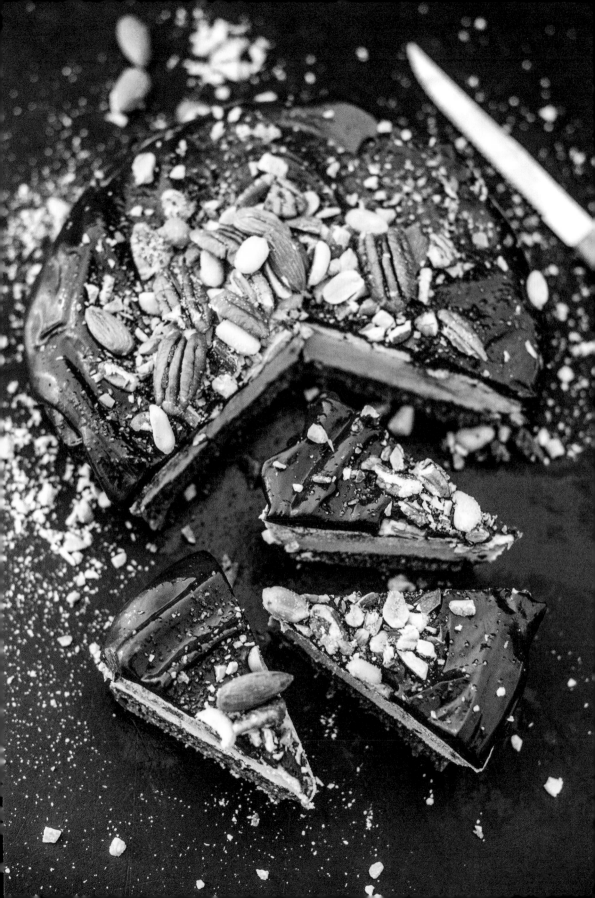

Thank You!

... to my parents, for always being there for me and for always supporting me on my way. I'm so incredibly thankful for everything and proud to have such wonderful parents. Mum and Dad, you're the best and you always will be!

... to the two very best roommates a girl could have, Fabia (my sister-heart) and Luisa. Thank you for tasting so many of my recipes during the past four months and for letting me turn the kitchen into my living room. I really appreciate your understanding!

... to the best friends in the world. My girls Alice, Sophia, Tanja, Sara, Andrea, Aita and Annigna. For your help on which pictures to choose (yes, you were literally bombarded with them), for your honesty, and for always motivating me and simply being there for me. I know that I can always count on you and I'm incredibly thankful for that!

... to Samira Meier, who shot the cover that I couldn't be happier with. And of course all the other pictures of me in the book. You're such a talented lady and know how to capture people in their most natural way. What more can I say than: 'Sam, you're the man!'

... to Roger, for the amazing logo and cover design. With your work and effort, you helped me to give *Eat Better Not Less* character and created exactly what I had in mind. Muito obrigado!

... to my management, especially Dominik, for your support, help and precious guidance with everything since we started working together. I wouldn't be where I am today and with your help my book is finally available in the English market.

... to Kevin and Sandra who helped me with the translation and proofreading of the English version and showed so much enthusiasm right from the start. You've honestly been such a big support and I'm so happy to have worked with you!

... to Aashika, whom I'm so happy and thankful to call my friend, advisor and secret sister. Thank you for teaching me to stay true to my work and myself (I just wanna be me, I wanna be free – you know it girl!) And of course for proofreading all the recipes!

... to all my other friends, my family members and acquaintances who supported me with motivating words and always showed a big interest in my work. You know who you are, so thank you, thank you, thank you!

... to all the brands and everybody who has supported me with products like superfoods, kitchen utensils and much, much more. You made it possible for me to create such a variety of recipes with the appropriate tools and to set the philosophy of *Eat Better Not Less* in pictures and scene.

... and last but most certainly not least, to YOU! To every single person who is reading this right now (yes, exactly, you)! To the ones who have supported me from the very beginning, who visit my blog daily, follow me on Instagram, Facebook or other social media, like and comment on the pictures. Your comments are what motivate me to keep doing what I do, get better and create recipes with the motto *Eat Better Not Less*, which should motivate and inspire you in turn, that a healthy and balanced diet and lifestyle is fun, enjoyable and doesn't have anything to do with restriction. Without you I would have never been able to write this cookbook; I wouldn't be who and where I am today. This journey has brought me so much, so many experiences from which I could learn and grow. I honestly can't thank you enough for that. All I hope and wish for is that I can give you back as much as possible with this book and that you, in turn, can be your very own artist in the kitchen. Like I said: everybody can cook. It's just something you have to practice and, most importantly, do with a lot of passion, imagination and creativity!

Thank you in every single language there is on this planet and all the others in this universe! THANK YOU!

xx Nadia

WEBSITE   www.eatbetternotless.com
INSTAGRAM   @nadiadamaso_ebnl
FACEBOOK   eatbetternotlessnadiadamaso
PINTEREST   nadiadamasoebnl
TWITTER   EBNLnadiadamaso

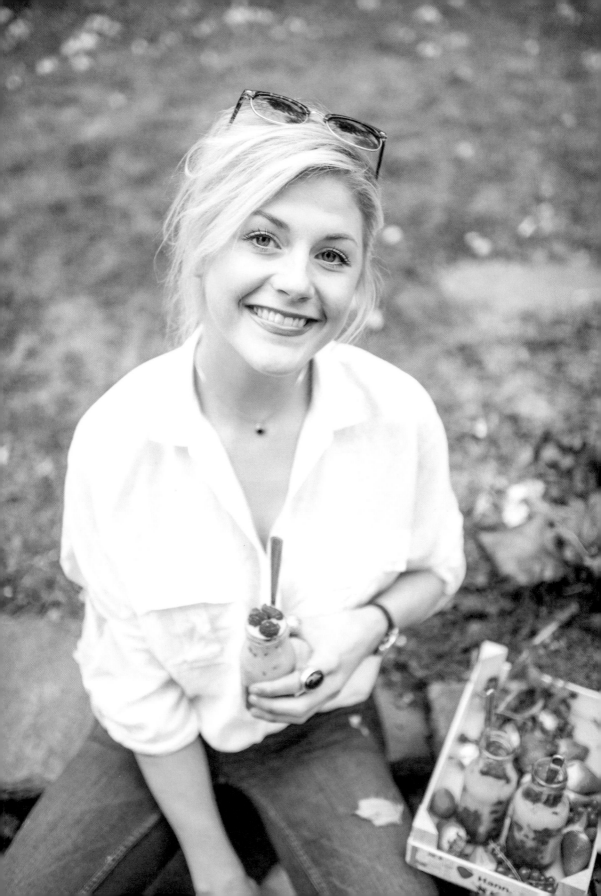

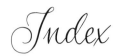

Index

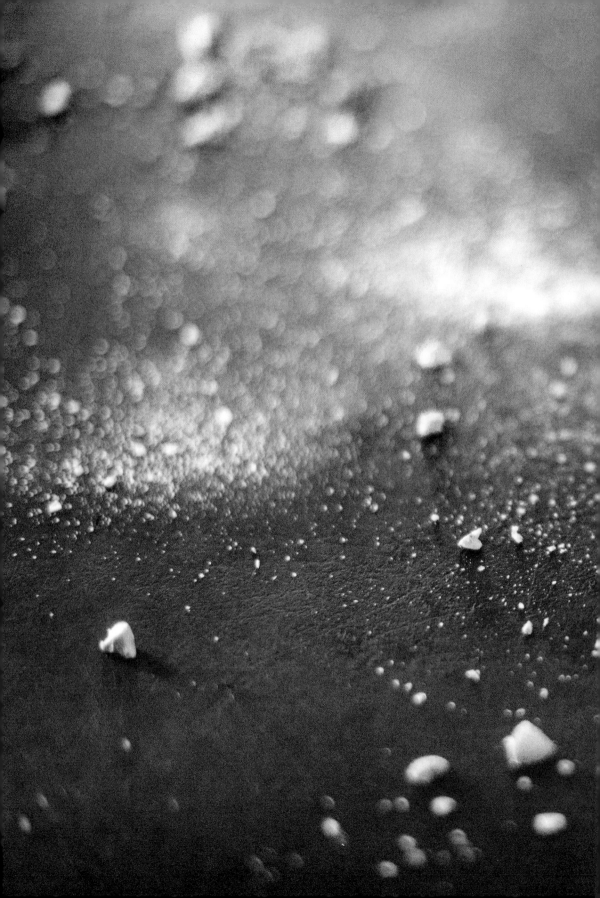